GOOD NEWS

FOR

BAD BACKS

GOOD NEWS
FOR
BAD BACKS

Robert L. Swezey, M.D.
Annette M. Swezey

Illustrations by Mary Benz Deckert

KNIGHTSBRIDGE PUBLISHING COMPANY
NEW YORK

DISCLAIMER

This book represents the authors' opinions and best advice to low back pain
sufferers. The guidelines that we give you to help assess your pain level and
determine appropriate treatment strategies are designed to inform you as to
what steps you can take to help relieve your back pain. The danger of self-
diagnosis and self-treatment is all too apparent. The information in this book
should be used in conjunction with the advice and consent of your physician. In
the final analysis, only your physician knows your case and can determine what
is best for you.

Copyright © 1990 by Robert L. Swezey and Annette M. Swezey

All rights reserved. Printed in the U.S.A.

Published in the United States by
Knightsbridge Publishing Company
255 East 49th Street
New York, New York 10017

Library of Congress Cataloging-in-Publication Data

Swezey, Robert L.
  Good news for bad backs / Robert L. Swezey and Annette M. Swezey.
—1st ed.
    p. cm.
  ISBN 1-877961-01-9 : $19.95
  1. Backache. 2. Backache—Exercise therapy. I. Swezey, Annette
M., 1928– . II. Title.
RD771.B217S94   1990
617.5'64062—dc20   90-31168
                                                        CIP

ISBN: 0-877961-01-9

Design by *Rem Studio*.

10 9 8 7 6 5 4 3 2 1

FIRST EDITION

To our beloved parents,
Dr. Samuel and Birdie Swezey,
and
Jack and Pauline Maler.
Without their love we would not be.
Without their caring we could not care
nor care to write
so that you may be helped.

CONTENTS

III. THE HEALTH CARE TEAM, DIAGNOSIS, AND TREATMENT

IV. ERGONOMICS: BACK PAIN PROTECTION AND PREVENTION

V. EXERCISE, FITNESS, AND FUN

LIST OF

ILLUSTRATIONS

ACKNOWLEDGMENTS

We would especially like to acknowledge our patients, who over the years have taught us so much and given us this knowledge that we can now share.

This book would not have come about without the guidance of James Preminger, who led us to Gerry Sindell. Gerry took our work, helped us organize it, and with the outstanding editorial contribution of Shelly Usen, made this book a reality. The day-in, day-out, page-by-page labor of putting this book on paper was done thoughtfully, tirelessly and, we think, lovingly, by Peggy Hughes. Mary Benz Deckert's art work speaks for itself and gives this book a special visual flavor. She has been an essential part of our team, working with us at The Arthritis & Back Pain Center to help create our patient-education hand-outs in the attractive, clear, graphic manner demonstrated in this book. It is our hope that the contributions of our patients and co-workers will be rewarded by the help that you can receive from this book. Thanks to all of you.

GOOD NEWS

FOR

BAD BACKS

INTRODUCTION

"I know just when I did it. Saturday I was trying to move the couch and I heard something go 'crack' in my back. I couldn't straighten up—it was so painful."

"I was doing a lot of work around the house over the weekend and naturally I felt a little achy. Then I stepped off the curb and—pow!"

"I've had a bad cold; I've been coughing and sneezing a lot, and this morning when I got up I had to crawl to the bathroom."

"I really don't know what caused it."

Unfortunately for many of us, one of these statements (or something similar) sounds all too familiar. We have become a part of the great host of adults who suffer from low back pain.

Good News for Bad Backs is for all present, past, and future back pain sufferers. This book is for you whether your back pain is mild, moderate, or severe. The *good news* is that this book can guide you to make the right choices concerning the cause, treatment, and prevention of low back pain, and it can help you put your back pain as far behind you as possible.

How good can a bad back be? Statistics show that ninety

percent of us, at some time or another, will have an episode of severe, disabling back pain. Fortunately, the majority (80%) will be out of that pain and back in action within a month—with or without treatment! The problem is that we can't tell initially if we're going to join the 80% who will get better no matter what, or the 20% who may be considerably less fortunate.

The *good news* is that most low back pain is preventable, and this book will show you how. More *good news* is that most low back pain can be successfully treated *without* surgery. That means that even if you're one of the unlucky twenty percent who do not recover in a month's time, there's a great likelihood that you can get over your back pain without resorting to heavy medication dosages or surgical procedures.

Knowing how to lie, sit, squat, and lift, and how to exercise to relieve pain and recondition injured and weakened back structures is what this book is about. By utilizing the back protection and prevention exercises that are featured in this book and used at our Arthritis & Back Pain Center in Santa Monica, California, back pain sufferers can find relief and enjoy a useful, productive, and fulfilling life. However, *Good News for Bad Backs* is not intended as a guide to self-diagnosis and self-treatment. It's a handy reference book that should help you understand what might be causing your low back pain, and it's a resource for some simple methods you can use to relieve your pain, to keep you from sliding backward, and to help you find the right path back to back health.

Good News for Bad Backs is divided into five parts. Part I—Anatomy and Diseases: The Ways and Means of Back Pain helps you to understand how your back is constructed, and what hurts and why, and the causes of back pain.

Part II—What's Wrong with Your Back and How to Fix It helps you to determine how severe your back pain problem is. You will then be able to make the right choices and the right decisions about medicines, therapy, exercise, and activities. Part II will help you choose the best ways to get back pain off your back.

Part III—The Health Care Team, Diagnosis, and Treatment helps you to find the right physician for your back pain problem, discusses what diagnosis he or she may make, and presents the various treatments available to you.

Part IV—Ergonomics: Back Pain Protection and Prevention

provides detailed instructions for performing activities without back strain, ranging from getting in and out of bed to household chores, driving, working, loving, traveling, and recreation. You will learn how to get on the right road back from back pain.

Part V—Exercise, Fitness, and Fun designates specific exercises designed to relieve pain, recondition your back, and help prevent future back pain. In addition, you will learn what sports and recreational activities are right for you, and how to safely participate in your chosen sports without having to back off with back pain.

You may first want to read about the anatomy of the back, or you may prefer to first learn about prevention or exercises or other treatments. However you choose to use this book, there is a great deal of good and useful news for you to explore and absorb in the way that works best for you. Practice the precepts of this book and there will be GOOD NEWS FOR YOUR BAD BACK!

I.

ANATOMY AND

DISEASES:

THE WAYS AND MEANS

OF BACK PAIN

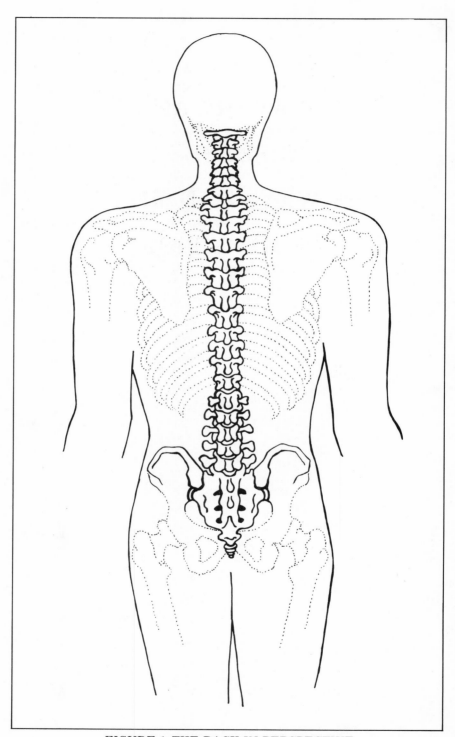

FIGURE 1 THE BACK IN PERSPECTIVE

1.

ANATOMY—

WHAT'S

BACK THERE?

The most common cause of low back pain, or lumbago as it's commonly been called, is a sprain or strain affecting the last two vertebrae of the lumbar spine.

Although this simple statement makes sense, in a way it does not really mean much, because most of us do not have a clear picture of our spinal anatomy. It shouldn't be too surprising that we know so little about our backs. First of all, unless we are contortionists, it is pretty hard to inspect our backs closely, even with the aid of mirrors! Secondly, the ratio of nerves sending messages about the goings-on in our backs compared to our fingertips or tongues is much less than a hundred to one. So, we get fewer messages and tend to ignore our backs, taking them for granted until something goes wrong and the back talks back!

SPINAL COLUMN

Let's get better acquainted with our backs. We can start at the top of our spinal column, or "backbone," secure in the knowledge that each of us, like all other mammals—including giraffes—

7

has seven back bones in the neck, called *cervical vertebrae* (a *vertebra* is one of the 24 back bones that are linked to form the bony vertebral or spinal column). These seven cervical vertebrae support the 12 pounds of skull and the delicate brain that it encloses.

Also included in the 24 vertebrae are 12 *thoracic* or *dorsal vertebrae* located in the back of the chest where the ribs attach. Finally, supporting the weight of the upper body, are the five low back or *lumbar vertebrae* that complete the 24-bone spinal column (*Figs. 2 and 3*).

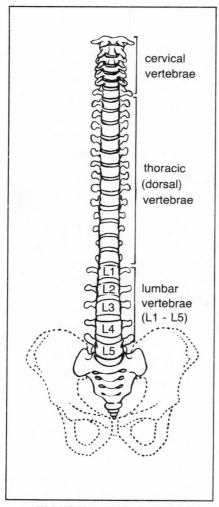

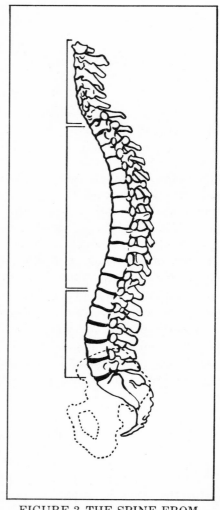

FIGURE 2 THE SPINE FROM
THE FRONT

FIGURE 3 THE SPINE FROM
THE SIDE

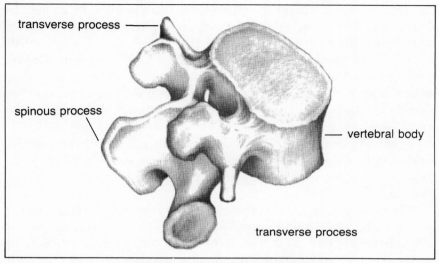

transverse process

spinous process

vertebral body

transverse process

FIGURE 4 LUMBAR VERTEBRA

Each vertebra in the spinal column consists of a main oval block-shaped bony structure called the *vertebral body* (*Fig. 4*). Attached to the back of the vertebral body is a bony arch that straddles and protects the spinal cord and nerves. On top of this sits the *spinous process*. The vertebral spinous processes are the bony bumps we can feel protruding from the back of our spine (try feeling them). Although many people assume that the spinous process is the actual vertebra or backbone, it is really just a large, bony strut that juts back from the vertebral body, much like a dorsal fin on a whale's back. In the lumbar area, the vertebral body and the shock-absorbing linkages, or *disks*, that separate one vertebra from another actually lie about two inches below the skin that covers the protruding tip of a spinous process.

On each side of the bony arch is a large, stubby, winglike projection called the *transverse process*. The spinous process, the bony arch, and the transverse processes provide attachments for the muscles that control spinal movements in a manner analogous to the effects of air currents on the tail and wings of an airplane.

SACRUM AND COCCYX

Joining with the five lumbar vertebrae are five fused vertebrae that comprise the *sacrum*, the bone that forms the back of the pelvis (*Fig. 5*). Nature, apparently, is indecisive about how to distribute these ten vertebrae. Although the usual division is 50:50 (five lumbar vertebrae and five fused sacral vertebrae), often the top sacral vertebra fails to fuse and forms what is called a "sixth" lumbar vertebra. Or, the fifth lumbar vertebra may fuse with the sacrum prior to birth, leaving only four movable lumbar vertebrae. *However, these variations rarely, if ever, cause back problems.*

Last but not least, we all have a little tail called the *coccyx*, hidden out of sight between our buttocks. It consists of three to five tiny vertebrae that are attached to the bottom tip of the sacrum.

The bony spinal or vertebral column is designed to anchor our muscles and support our vital organs so that we can stand erect, breathe, eat, walk, lie, jump, twist, lift, climb, or sit with minimal effort and maximal resiliency. It also shelters the delicate spinal cord and the nerves that branch out from it. No wonder we think so little of a spineless person!

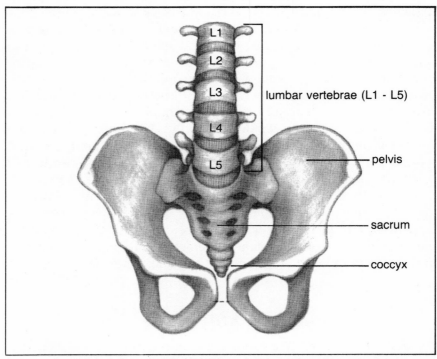

FIGURE 5 LUMBAR-PELVIC AREA FROM THE FRONT

THE SPINAL NERVES AND WHERE
THE NERVES EMERGE

The *spinal cord* is like a long tail of nerve tissue hanging down from beneath the brain. It is sheltered by the bony spinal column and by delicate membranes that create a tube filled with a watery spinal fluid in which the spinal cord and nerves are floated for added protection. The spinal cord consists of layers of delicate nerve cells and nerve fibers that relay messages from the brain to the body and vice versa. The entire length of the spinal cord is protected by the disks and the vertebral bodies in front, and by the bony arches, ligaments, and facet joints in back (*see pg. 14; Fig. 9*). At the level of each lumbar disk a pair of spinal nerves branch off from the spinal cord and travel out through a tunnel formed by the disk below and the facet joint above. Each spinal nerve consists of a bundle of tiny wirelike fibers that transmit messages to and from the brain and spinal cord to various parts of the body. A small branch of the nerve leads to the back and a larger branch to a specified region of skin, muscles, and body organs.

The large branches of the fourth and fifth spinal nerves emerge at the fourth and fifth lumbar disks, L4 and L5 (*see Fig. 5, pg. 10*), and join with the first two nerves emerging at the sacrum, S1 and S2, to form the *sciatic nerve* (*Fig. 6*). If you sprain your ankle, a message travels along the sciatic nerve to the spinal cord and to the brain. In a flash, you will be painfully aware of what's happened, but before you realize it, the brain will already have transmitted messages down the spinal cord and out through the spinal nerves to the leg, to help you limp away. If, on the other hand, you wrench your back and sprain the fifth lumbar disk, the swollen bulging disk can pinch and irritate the fifth spinal nerve before the nerve separates into its branches to the back and to the sciatic nerve. This will send messages to both your back and your leg. Now you have back pain (*lumbago*) and leg pain (*sciatica*).

THE DISKS AND THE BONES OF CONTENTION
IN LOW BACK PAIN

Between each vertebral body and between the last lumbar vertebra and the sacrum, nature has supplied us with the shock-absorbing linkages called the *intervertebral* (between the verte-

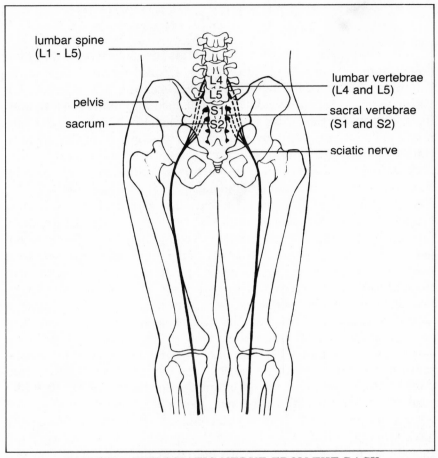

lumbar spine
(L1 - L5)

L4
L5
S1
S2

pelvis

sacrum

lumbar vertebrae
(L4 and L5)

sacral vertebrae
(S1 and S2)

sciatic nerve

FIGURE 6 THE SCIATIC NERVE FROM THE BACK

brae) *disks* (*Fig. 7*). The intervertebral disk fills an oval-shaped area about a quarter-inch thick that separates the bodies of two adjacent vertebrae. Many people mistakenly perceive the disk as popping in and out, like a washer or a computer disk; hence, a "slipped disk." In fact, the intervertebral disk consists of circular layers of tough fibrous ligaments that ring the upper and lower rims of each vertebral body. This fibrous ring of ligaments, called the *annulus* (ring) *fibrosus*, binds the vertebra above to the one below, creating the boundaries of and comprising the intervertebral joint. The annulus fibrosus encircles and contains the gooey *nucleus* (center) *pulposus* (pulpy), which has the consistency of thick wet paper pulp and which lubricates and nourishes the

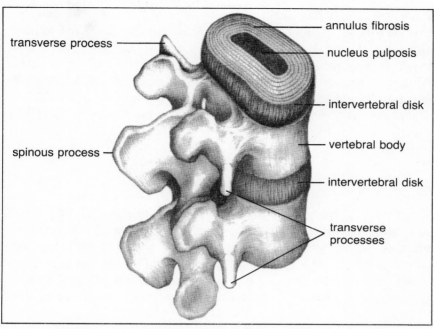

FIGURE 7 LUMBAR VERTEBRAE AND NORMAL DISK

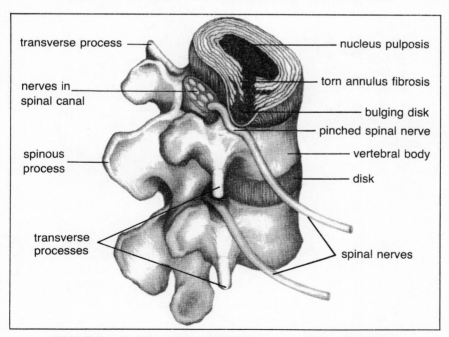

FIGURE 8 LUMBAR VERTEBRAE AND BULGING DISK

inner surface of the disk and acts as a shock absorber between the vertebrae. It is obvious, then, that the disk does not actually slip, but it can bulge (*Fig. 8*) and even tear so that a fragment is separated from the annulus into the vertebral canal. Clearly a broken fragment of the annulus is not something that can be slipped back into place, and we'll learn more about that when we read about what's out when the back goes out in Chapter 14.

FACET JOINTS

From both sides of the back of the vertebral arches, small, flat, bony "arms" project upward and interlock with similar downward directed "arms" from the vertebra above to form the *facet joints* (*Fig. 9*). The facet joints, which are about the size of the small joints in our fingers, serve to keep the vertebrae aligned as we bend and twist. (The smooth, shiny, hard, cartilage-covered

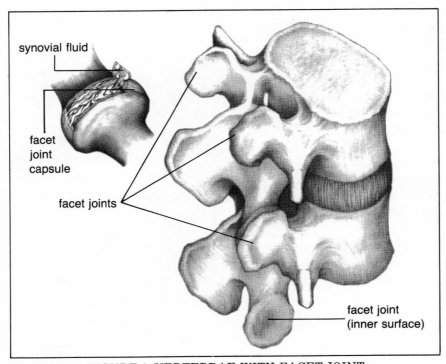

synovial fluid

facet joint capsule

facet joints

facet joint (inner surface)

FIGURE 9 VERTEBRAE WITH FACET JOINT

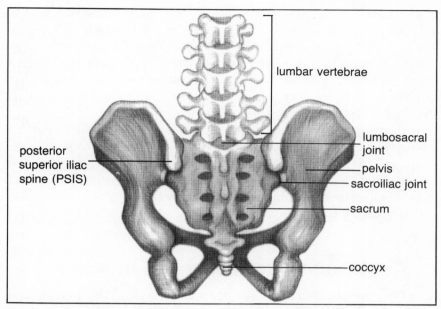

lumbar vertebrae

lumbosacral joint

posterior superior iliac spine (PSIS)

pelvis

sacroiliac joint

sacrum

coccyx

FIGURE 10 LUMBAR-PELVIC AREA FROM THE BACK

inner surface of these joints resembles the facets of cut stones; hence the name "facet joints.") The facet joints are bound together at their edges by tough ligaments called the *joint capsule*. The inner surface of the joint capsule has a smooth lining layer called the *synovium*, which produces *synovial fluid*, a fluid of syruplike consistency that lubricates and nourishes the joint surfaces.

There are also a number of other smaller and larger ligaments that connect various bony parts of one vertebra to those of the next. They help to protect the spinal cord and spinal nerves where there are gaps between the bony surfaces of the vertebrae, and they restrain potentially damaging spinal motion or, in fact, become sprained when excessive motion occurs.

THE SACROILIAC JOINTS

The *sacroiliac* (SI) *joints* are large, barely movable joints that connect the sacrum to the *iliac* bones, which form the sides of the pelvis. The outer sides of the iliac bones are shaped to serve as sockets for the hip joints. You can find the general area of the sacroiliac joints by feeling for two hard bony lumps that are the back ends of the iliac bones on either side (*Fig. 10*). These bony lumps (called the *posterior superior iliac spines*— PSIS) are located at the very back of the pelvis, about four inches apart, and are separated by the flat surface of the sacrum that lies between them. The actual sacroiliac joints are located about two inches anterior to these bony lumps.

Years ago, doctors thought most low back pain occurred when the sacroiliac joints slipped out of place. Although such slippage can occur when major injuries cause a tearing of the very strong ligaments that hold these joints together, sacroiliac joint displacement or malalignment is actually quite uncommon and is unlikely to cause pain or sciatica.

LIGAMENTS, TENDONS, AND MUSCLES

The vertebral column (along with the ribs, the pelvis, and the arm and leg bones) serves as a framework for the attachment of muscles. The framework of bones is held together with *ligaments*, fibrous tissues that resemble elastic bands in varying degrees of thickness and suppleness. Some of these ligaments are very firm and tough, while others are more delicate and supple. Each ligament is engineered to serve a specific purpose, binding one vertebra to the next while permitting modest movement in some planes but not others; or more rigidly, supporting the pelvis and its sacroiliac joints. The wrong move at the wrong time may cause injury or sprain of any of these ligaments. Typically, when this occurs, we experience back pain, which feels muscular. Indeed, if the pain is severe enough, the muscles will become rigidly tightened in a painful spasm that can prevent any motion. This reflex phenomenon is nature's way of causing the muscles to tighten and splint the body against any movement that might aggravate the injured area.

The real "shakers and movers" of the body are the *muscles*. No undulating belly dancer could even budge without the action of muscles. Muscles come in a variety of sizes and shapes, each designed to do a specific job. Large bulky muscles run the length of the spinal column, and very small muscles bridge from one vertebra to the next. Each muscle has its specific task and all muscles work in concert with each other. At any time, a given

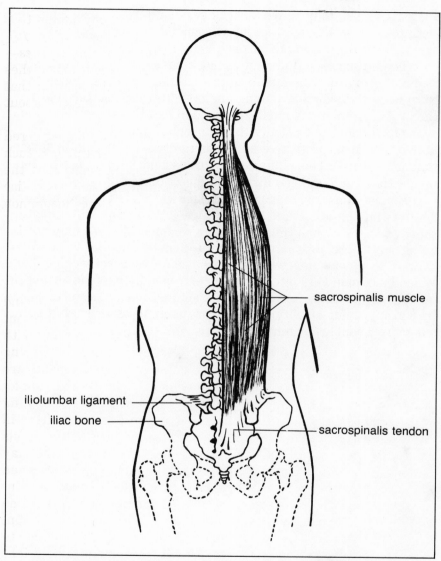

sacrospinalis muscle

iliolumbar ligament

iliac bone

sacrospinalis tendon

FIGURE 11 SPINAL MUSCLES, TENDONS, AND LIGAMENTS

muscle may be forcibly tightened, semi-relaxed but on hold, or completely relaxed, while muscles on the opposite side of the body may be vigorously contracting.

All muscles must attach to adjacent skeletal structures, and where they do so, the muscle merges into a band of fibrous tissues, similar to a ligament, called a *tendon*. Some tendons, such as those that move our fingers and toes, are long and stringlike, but the tendons of the spinal muscles typically are short, thick fibrous bands at each end of the muscle.

The muscles contain many small contractile fibers that, when stimulated by messages transmitted through nerves, cause them to tighten and shorten, pulling one bone toward another and thus causing movement. A muscle or tendon can be over-strained and cause back pain, but usually the "muscular" pain we feel is attributable to a firm, protective muscular tightening, or painful spasm, that occurs as a consequence of strains and sprains of the ligaments that surround the disks and facet joints.

Bones, muscles, nerves, and sinews hold us together and keep us on the go. That's when all goes well. But unfortunately there are times when things don't go so smoothly. We may not be going anywhere; we may be in a stop-and-go mode; we may be slowed to a walk; or we may even come to a screeching halt. When back pain gets into the picture, it usually gets our attention quickly. Sometimes, however, the back just makes peculiar noises that also get our attention and worry us unnecessarily. Let's find out more about what hurts and why.

2.

WHAT HURTS

AND WHY?

"OW!" That's probably the first sound you'll hear when back pain strikes, but it's not necessarily the only sound that back pain can elicit. In fact, there are a lot of nonverbal noises that can issue from the back. Some of them are signals of trouble and some are normal occurrences. What is the noise that's going on behind your back?

NOISE MAKERS IN THE BACK ROW

"Something just popped in my back!" It's enough to have back pain, without having to hear about it when you change positions or do your exercises. What is all that noise back there? It used to be attributable to a "crack in the sacroiliac." Whatever it is, *you* usually hear it louder than anyone else because your bones transmit sound better than the air around you. Your back, and even more so, your neck, shoulders, or knees may be creaking, cracking and at times popping, but you usually only notice these sounds when it is quiet, or on occasions when the noise is especially loud.

Creaking noises (doctors call this *crepitation*), which can be produced consistently by certain motions such as twisting your neck or shrugging your shoulders, are attributable to hard connective tissue, tendons, ligaments, or surrounding muscles rubbing against each other or against adjacent bone. Dry tissue within older and worn disks may also account for some of the creaking sounds that occur with twisting motions of the spine.

Leathery, coarse grating sounds are more apt to occur when thickened tendons rub against each other or adjacent bone. These sounds are most likely heard between the shoulder blades and the chest wall or in the shoulder joints, wrists, and knees. If there is no associated pain, there is really nothing to worry about.

Clicks, like cracking, are due to the movement of relatively dry disk material or small ligaments and muscles snapping over minor bony projections at facet joints or disk margins. These noises become more noticeable when age and wear-and-tear changes in these structures have taken their toll, but they have no significance in terms of what's causing your pain or whether or not you will get better. They're a little like the small bony outgrowths called *osteophytes* seen on X-rays of the spine—they tell you you've got some abnormalities back there, but they don't tell you if they're serious or even important to your present condition (*see* "*How About Tests for Arthritis?*" *pg. 109*). In fact, they will still be there if you should by chance have X-rays when your back is no longer hurting.

What about clunks and thuds? A thud in the back can be disconcerting. Usually this means that a larger ligament just snapped over a bony prominence. This is very common in the hip joints, where a twisting of the leg outward can snap the heavy ligament in front of the hip joint. Twisting it inward can snap a strong tendon over the outer bony prominence (the greater *trochanter*) on your thigh. These noises can be so loud that a hip dislocation is feared.

Finally, the pops and cracks can startle you or comfort you depending on whether or not they are perceived as a threatening noise, attributable to the spine being dislocated, or a friendly sound that signals a successful outcome of your favorite twisting maneuver. Many of the pops and cracking sounds (often called "audibles" by chiropractors) are louder versions of clicks and clunks. When a sound can only be made during one precise movement and is not reproducible for 10 to 30 minutes, this sound can be attributed to a sudden opening or gapping of a facet joint and is similar to the sound made when you crack your knuckles. The cracking sound is caused by water, bound in the joint lining, suddenly exploding into the vacuum created during the sudden gapping of the joint. The lag of 10 to 30 minutes before the joint can be re-popped is the time required for joint capsules to reabsorb the water so as to be primed for the next pop.

Now that we've considered some of the incidental background noises that can occur in normal backs, or in backs with minor but painless abnormalities, let's now look at the various ways in which back disorders cause pain and disability.

STRAINS AND SPRAINS

We said that the most common cause (about 95%) of low back pain is a strain or sprain in the ligaments between the fourth and fifth lumbar vertebrae. The term *strain* actually has several meanings. It is used to describe a vigorous effort, an overworked muscle, or a minor (micro) tear in a ligament, muscle, or tendon.

The term *sprain* means an actual gross tear in a ligament. Unfortunately, most of us have experienced a sprained ankle ligament. When the annulus fibrosus ligaments, which surround the disks, or the ligaments connecting the vertebrae or the facet joints are over-stressed, they will tear. Sprains (gross tears) and strains (micro tears) are particularly likely to occur when we are bending or lifting, and especially when we are bending, lifting, and twisting simultaneously. A tear or sprain of the annulus fibrosus, like that of any other ligament, causes local swelling and bruising. A minor sprain that affects primarily the inner fibers of the annulus fibrosus where there are no nerve endings can go unnoticed. But if the tear and swelling occur in the other fibers, the pain-sensitive nerve endings there will give us the message: We now have a backache.

BULGING DISKS AND NATURE'S BATTLE OF THE BULGE

When physicians talk about disk problems, they may choose to call it *discogenic disease, disk protrusion* or *herniation* (disk bulging), or *disk extrusion* (an actual tear through the annulus fibrosus, which allows some of the inner disk contents to intrude into the spinal canal, causing pressure on delicate nerves; *see Fig. 8, pg. 13*). Any way you say it—when you are fighting a bulging disk, it can mean trouble.

Delayed action: Often after a moderate and sometimes unnoted back strain, we get an uneasy feeling in our back, perhaps with some stiffness and the sense that all is not right. The discomfort may go away in a day or so, but sometimes during an ordinary activity, such as getting out of a chair, or sneezing, or bending over to tie shoes, we get—POW—back pain! What causes this back pain fuse to burn slowly and then explode? Sprains of the annulus fibrosus portion of the disk, unlike sprains elsewhere, often cause relatively little pain at first. Hours, and sometimes days, pass before the repeated stresses and strains of normal activity aggravate the initial injury and cause enough irritation and swelling to stimulate the pain fibers in the outer portion of the annulus fibrosus. Then we experience the pain and the muscle spasm that so often accompanies it.

The normal disk interior (the nucleus pulposus) has no blood circulation and therefore depends on seepage of body fluids through the annulus fibrosus for its nutrition. During the night, when we are lying down and when gravity is not causing the weight of the body to press on the disks, water is more readily absorbed into the nucleus pulposus. The disks actually become so bloated overnight that when we get up in the morning we are taller than we were when we went to bed the night before. In the instance of a sprained annulus fibrosus, it is common for the pain to go unnoted until the morning (or several mornings) after the injury, when normal overnight disk swelling and swelling due to the injury and to the added strains from daily activity combine to stretch the sensitive torn annulus fibrosus ligaments and stimulate the pain fibers. When this occurs we get the delayed bad news: lumbago—back pain!

LUMBAGO AND MUSCLE SPASM

So lumbago, in the vast majority of cases, is lumbar pain brought on by a strain or sprain of a lumbar disk and/or facet joint between L4 and L5 or L5 and S1 (*see Fig. 6, pg. 12*).

Accompanying this strain, some—and occasionally all—of the muscles in the low back and/or the buttocks may undergo a prolonged, painful contraction or spasm. Sometimes the muscles of the back and buttocks are actually strained, which means that the muscles themselves are injured, and this too can cause a painful muscle contraction or spasm.

PUTTING YOUR FINGER ON THE PAIN: TRIGGER POINTS, TENDER POINTS, BURSITIS, AND FIBROMYALGIA

Typically, only a small portion of a muscle contracts, as an apparent protective response to a disk or facet strain or sprain, forming a tender knot that you can feel. These partial muscle spasms apparently protect you from trying activities that are too vigorous, but still permit you to get around—albeit not comfortably. When these knots are stroked, a visible contraction can sometimes be seen or felt. This can be accompanied by a shooting radiating pain, hence the name *trigger point*.

Although trigger points are tender, there are other types of tender points that commonly accompany low back pain. It is not clear why certain areas of muscle attachment commonly become irritated during the course of back pain (this also occurs in the neck and shoulders when disks in the neck are affected). In the case of irritation of a muscle-bone attachment, one can postulate that a strained and contracted muscle may be pulling excessively hard against its bony attachment, causing a tender point of irritation—such as the pain and tenderness of the strained muscle attachments at the elbow in "tennis elbow." Whether this is the case, or whether the irritation or tenderness is due to a reflex phenomenon similar to that which causes trigger points, we simply do not know. What we do know is that treatments used for trigger points are often helpful in relieving the pain and tenderness in tender points as well.

Another type of tender point is also common, but is frequently overlooked. The body has a number of *bursae*, little flat sacks that manufacture a small amount of synovial (joint) fluid to reduce friction caused by certain muscles rubbing against each other or against bone. The best known bursa in the body overlies the shoulder joint, but there are a number of these bursae situated around the hips and buttocks and elsewhere. Perhaps the idea of someone lying down or hobbling around with back pain getting an irritated bursa or *bursitis*—a disorder we associate with excessive activity—just doesn't sound right. Nonetheless, bursitis associated with low back pain is common and occasionally disabling. Bursitis, like other tender points that can develop despite the absence of vigorous activity and overuse, probably arises from back-pain-stimulated reflexes that cause blood vessel congestion, swelling, and irritation of the bursa.

Some patients seem to be inordinately susceptible to the development of trigger points and tender points. When this occurs, we say that they have *fibrositis*—irritation of the connecting tissues between muscles and muscle attachments to bone. Or we may call it *fibromyalgia*—pain in muscles and tender points. "What Else Could Be Going On Back There?" in Chapter 3 (*see pg. 27*) will help you decide if fibrositis is something that might be of concern to you.

SCIATICA

If a branch of the sciatic nerve gets "pinched," causing pressure on the nerve, we get *sciatica*, or leg pain. Sciatica occurs when the nerve is pinched, either by a swollen, bulging disk in front; by swelling of the ligaments behind the facet joint; by a fragment of the interior or outer portion of a disk that has broken through or off of the annulus fibrosus and has entered the spinal canal; or by a combination of these factors.

We can now see that the back is a finely engineered structure capable of providing rigid support to the body as well as supple and graceful movement. The vertebrae serve as the bridgework of the back and are separated by shock-absorbing disks, which are tied together with strategically placed ligaments. Spinal movement occurs through careful orchestrated muscular actions that are directed by messages transmitted through the spinal cord and nerves. This engineering marvel, like all structures, can have small imperfections that make it vulnerable to strain, or it can be caused to function in ways that exceed its design constraints. The resulting strains, sprains, and pains are the usual disorders that bring us to the doctor. Let's find out more about the mechanical disorders of our spinal structures, how we diagnose them, and what we can do about them.

3.

WHAT TO

WORRY ABOUT:

BACK PAIN

DANGER SIGNALS

Although most low back and sciatic problems are caused by injury to the disks and/or the facet joints, by no means are all back pains attributable to these structures. Most disk-related problems, sprains, and strains, if given proper care, will heal themselves. We worry because we are afraid that a disk problem means severe disability and possible surgery. We also worry when our back aches and we do not know what is causing it, how long it will last, or what is going to happen next. We worry that our back pain may be due to cancer, crippling arthritis, or other serious disease.

Many patients know precisely how their back strain occurred and are primarily concerned with getting rid of the pain. But since it is not unusual for disks to swell painlessly for several days after an injury and only then begin to cause noticeable pain or lingering soreness, a lot of us are unaware of the exact cause of the injury to our backs. In fact, we usually pay so little attention to how we use our backs, it is a wonder that they tolerate such a beating before finally letting us know how badly we are abusing them. Pulling weeds, packing, cleaning the garage, filing, sneezing, trying on clothes, aerobic dancing, unloading the car, jogging, driving, scrubbing floors; these activities are nothing unusual . . . until that last time—then we have low back pain to worry about!

When the low back pain begins with no apparent cause, so do the worries. The more severe the pain, the more it can worry us, and rightly so. But if the pain is very severe and comes on rapidly, the chances are it can be attributed to a disk sprain and will go away in a few days or weeks. If, on the other hand, your back pain has any of the Danger Signals listed below, then the chances are greater that you have something more serious to worry about, and you should see your doctor to find out what is wrong.

DANGER SIGNALS

1. Pain with no obvious cause
2. Pain gradual in onset and increasing in severity
3. Pain lasting more than three weeks
4. Pain and weakness or numbness in a leg
5. Pain unrelieved by rest, pain at night, pain for which there is no comfortable position
6. Pain and sickness, fever, chills, sweats, loss of appetite, nausea, weight loss
7. Pain and kidney or bladder dysfunction
8. Pain and constipation, diarrhea, or incontinence

HELP YOUR DOCTOR—DON'T BACK OFF

Most of us hate to bother the doctor or make a big deal out of minor ills. Nonetheless, pain that interferes with our ability to live normally gets our attention and demands prompt relief, or at least a decent explanation.

There is a classic gag about diagnosis in dermatology: "What do you think this rash is, doc?" "Had it before?" "Yep." "Well, looks like you've got it again!" The parallel in back pain is all too obvious. If it hurt like this before and it is hurting now, it is probably the same old back pain—whatever it is. In fact, most of us have minor aches and pains that go away with no treatment, or as a result of—or even in spite of—our favorite remedies. By and large, if you know how you hurt your back, can tolerate the discomfort with nothing much more than aspirin or rest, and are improving each day since it started, you can safely avoid visiting your doctor. But if the pain is so severe that you need a strong pain pill, or if you really don't know why you are hurting, it is best to at least explain your symptoms to the doctor and let him or her plan with you what the next step should be—whether it's "Stay in bed for two days," "Come over to the office right now," or "Stop your aerobic dancing for one week." If an illness like a severe back strain or a heart attack strikes suddenly and dramatically, we usually try and find out what it is and begin treatment promptly. But if it is gradual in onset with only mild, vague symptoms—"I don't feel right; maybe I am over-tired, or catching a cold, or maybe I have kidney trouble or mild back strain"—it may take longer for us to decide that we are not quite well and that we should see a physician, a medical doctor, to find out why (*see Chapter 12*).

WHAT ELSE COULD BE GOING ON BACK THERE?

If you are young and healthy, and particularly if you are a male and have persistent low back pain, the possibility of an arthritic disorder, which runs in families and is called *ankylosing spondylitis*, should be considered. See your doctor. If you are a young female, gynecological problems are not uncommon causes of back pain. See your doctor. Rarely, bacteria will settle in the disk and cause an infection; and in some parts of the world, tuberculosis and undulent fever (*brucellosis*) can infect the spine, but this is extraordinarily rare for those who are apt to be readers of this book. Kidney infections or painful passing of a kidney stone at any age can cause back pain, and this is usually associated with blood or pus in the urine. Typically, this type of pain is unrelieved by rest, and if there is infection in the kidney or bladder, there is usually an urgency to urinate, often associated with a fever or a sick sensation. See your doctor.

As we get older, the disorders associated with advancing years are more apt to enter the picture—but they are rarely responsible for back pain in someone who feels well and gets relief by lying down. In men, prostatic infections, enlargements, and tumors are occasionally responsible for low back pain. In rare cases, a major artery will develop a weak spot, called an *aneurysm*, and each pulse will cause blood to rush into the ballooning, thinned-out blood vessel wall, creating a pressure-pain on the structures adjacent to the spine. This is an extremely rare cause of steady or pulsating back pain and usually occurs in patients with high blood pressure and hardening of the arteries. If neglected, the aneurysm can burst, and this can result in a fatal hemorrhage. You probably do not have this problem, but if you suspect it and have not done so already—see your doctor.

Another disorder that occurs in older patients (past 50), which affects the shoulders and hips with a severe stiffness and aching, is called *polymyalgia rheumatica* (many muscle aches). This disorder is often associated with weakness, fatigue, and loss of appetite; sometimes with fever; and less commonly, with a peculiar chronic inflammation of the small arteries, especially in the scalp and, more seriously, affecting the eye and other vital structures. Patients with this disorder have a very high rate of sedimentation of their blood (*elevated sed rate*) and usually are cured with cortisone-like drugs in low doses, but this requires physician-supervised treatment for many months in order to avoid complications and recurrences.

It is no secret that various kinds of cancers occur more commonly as we grow older. Some of these originate in bones, in the bone marrow, or in the spinal canal. Some cancers spread into the bone from adjacent structures like the prostate gland. Some are spread around the body in the bloodstream, becoming lodged and growing in bone, originating from such remote sites as the breasts, kidneys, lungs, or thyroid gland. Obviously, these are extremely serious problems and require anticancer therapy. Your doctor can help you find out if cancer is present, so it can be treated.

OSTEOPOROSIS

One of the most common painful back disorders (but rarely a cause of low back pain) occurs most commonly in postmenopausal women and is attributable to *osteoporosis*. Osteoporosis means porous bone and is ordinarily due to a combination of things: a relative reduction of female hormones, which normally help retain calcium in the bone; a previously low calcium diet; and lack of exercise. It is much more commonly a problem in women who are light complected, small, and slender, with delicate bone structures. Osteoporosis leads to fractures of wrists, hips, ribs, and of the upper spine, but rarely does it cause fractures or symptoms in the low back. In fact, in patients with low back pain and osteoporosis, a so-called "spontaneous" *low* lumbar vertebral fracture should suggest to your doctor that the problem is more complicated and that an associated malignancy has to be considered. Since osteoporosis is a disorder of calcium metabolism, it will be worsened by poor general nutrition and a lack of calcium and vitamin D. It may also be caused by disorders of the thyroid and parathyroid glands; by poor absorption of calcium due to liver, kidney, and bowel disorders; or as a consequence of medication affecting calcium absorption —particularly cathartics and certain aluminum-containing antacid drugs (not to mention smoking and alcohol abuse).

If you have osteoporosis, the proper combination of diet, exercise, and medication, to prevent its worsening, should be determined by your doctor.

GOUT

Disorders of calcium metabolism and thyroid dysfunction are called *metabolic disorders*. One such metabolic disorder often accused falsely of causing back pain is *gout*. Gout is due to an excessive accumulation of a natural substance, a metabolite called *uric acid*, in the body. Whereas deposits of uric acid crystals typically cause severe arthritis in the big toe and in other joints, they almost never cause an arthritis flare-up in the spine. Unfortunately, patients with back pain often take aspirin and/or a few drinks for relief, and this can temporarily raise the level of uric acid in the blood. This may cause the unsophisticated physician to suspect that the high uric acid has caused gout and back pain. If gout has been your back pain diagnosis—get a second opinion from a rheumatologist (arthritis specialist) before you spend the rest of your life taking pills for a gouty condition that you may not have. Doubt gout if your back is out!

WHAT ELSE CAN CAUSE LOW BACK PAIN?

Whenever a patient asks, "Is it possible that _____ can cause _____?" the answer is always, "Yes," because in medicine, almost anything is possible. But let's be reasonable and practical. Since rare or one-time-only happenings are just that—we shall try and stay with what is common and can therefore reasonably be suspected as a cause of your low back pain.

DISH

There is a condition, associated with some loss of spinal motion but not an actual feeling of stiffness, which is often confused with *osteoarthritis* of the spine. In this disorder, the disks are not damaged, but for unknown reasons, bone is laid down in the normal non-bony fibrous ligaments that surround the disks. Obviously, with bone bridging from one vertebra to the next, there can be no motion between the vertebrae. The patient is aware of a lack of suppleness but otherwise feels no discomfort. X-rays in these patients often show a massive extra bone formation that is frequently incorrectly interpreted as severe arthritis. If you have some stiffness of your spine but minimal or no aches and pains in your back, are past 50 years of age, and have been told that you have terrible arthritis in your spine— get another medical opinion. You may have DISH, which stands for *disseminated* (all over the place) *idiopathic* (don't know what causes it) *skeletal* (skeletal) *hyperostosis* (too much bone). If you do have DISH, even though there is no way to treat it, you really need not worry about it.

SPONDYLOLISTHESIS

Some children develop a weakening of the support struts that attach the facet joints to the vertebrae. Later in life this weak area, called a *spondylolysis* (spine defect), gives way, and part of one vertebra slips forward over the vertebra below. This slippage, called a *spondylolisthesis* (spine slippage), can be a predisposing cause of back strain and pain. A spondylolisthesis can also occur when the disk deteriorates, and instead of the two adjacent vertebrae just jamming closer together, weakened ligaments may allow one vertebra to partially override the other. This too can cause back strain in the facet joints and secondary wear-and-tear arthritis or osteoarthritis in these joints.

SPINAL STENOSIS

When one vertebra slips forward or backward out of alignment, it may squeeze the spinal nerve roots. If the carefully protected tunnel through which the nerve roots pass happens to be a narrow one or is made smaller by a bulging disk or bony enlargement around the disk that is secondary to osteoarthritis, or if the ligaments are thickened in these areas, the spinal canal is said to be *stenosed*, or narrowed. This condition, called *spinal stenosis*, may be associated with back pain, but usually does not cause severe back discomfort per se. Rather, when a person with spinal stenosis stands or walks, he gets increasing heaviness and possibly weakness and numbness in his legs, which is relieved promptly by bending forward, sitting, or lying. The weakness is due to squeezing of the spinal nerves, which can be aggravated in spondylolisthesis when the vertebrae slip one over the other while we are standing erect. It is important to know that most patients with spinal stenosis or with spondylolisthesis have no symptoms whatsoever, and those with symptoms can usually be treated without surgery. Still, these are more complicated disorders and, particularly in the case of spinal stenosis, are often confused with circulatory problems because of the weakness and/or pain that comes on after walking short distances—so you need your doctor, and probably an orthopedic or neurosurgical specialist as well, to help you sort this out.

SERIOUS SCIATICA AND PINCHED NERVES

There is one last group of problems associated with low back pain that is clearly worth worrying about, and that is low back pain with loss of strength or sensation—which is due to *sciatic nerve pinching*. Even more important is any difficulty in bowel, bladder, or sexual function associated with back pain. Any suspected impairment of the bladder, of the bowel, or of sexual function associated with back pain constitutes a potential surgical emergency, as permanent damage to the delicate nerves that supply these vital organs can occur rapidly. Consult your physician immediately.

Weakness or numbness in a leg or foot (which is caused by a bulging disk and results from a pinching of a branch of the sciatic nerve—*see Fig. 8, pg. 13*) requires prompt attention, but it is not necessarily emergent unless it is rapidly progressive. In the vast majority of such cases, these symptoms improve with rest and proper treatment, and surgery is not required. Nevertheless, your doctor should be promptly contacted in the presence of such symptoms.

FIBROSITIS AND MYOFASCIAL PAIN

There is a disorder that can worry you and usually does, and the more you worry the worse it gets. It is most commonly called *fibrositis*, but there is no "itis" or inflammation, and it mostly affects muscles, not fibrous tissue. It is also called *fibromyositis*, but there is no inflammation in the muscles either. It has been less commonly called *myofascial pain*, or *fibromyalgia*, which probably gets closer to what it is—an aching (*algia*) of muscles and connective tissue around the muscles. Another name, even less commonly used, is *myogelosis*—which describes the peculiar knotlike muscle swelling (*myo* = muscle; *gel* = firm swelling) in muscles that, when pressed, may refer pain to other nearby and sometimes distant regions—so-called trigger points. For example, a "trigger" in the *gluteus medius* muscle (which lies above the hip on the outer side of the pelvis), when pressed, can "shoot" pain down the outside of the leg to the knee and may mimic sciatic pain.

Most patients with disk and facet joint problems develop some fibrositic trigger points. This seems to be a natural response of the body—maybe nature stirs up these painful areas of spasm in the muscles to keep us from doing more harm to our backs. They seem to be there to say, "Don't overdo it, because all is not well back there." But oftentimes these trigger points seem to send out too strong a message, and a vicious cycle gets established. The message from the source of trouble in the spine to the trigger point gets so well grooved that the soreness in the trigger point becomes a new satellite message center rather than just the relay point it was intended to be. Now the trigger is sending messages to the spinal cord that there is a sore spot in the buttocks (or wherever the trigger point happens to be), and the message center sends a message back to the trigger point—hang in there, stay in spasm even if it hurts! When this occurs, and we are no longer hurting for any good reason, treatment of a trigger point alone may relieve the back problem or a referred sciatic-like pain.

In some unfortunate people, a disk injury may be the beginning of a chronic state of hyperirritability of these trigger points. Each trigger point that becomes painful can stimulate new trigger points to help protect against the pain coming from the original trigger point. Such a patient is like a pinball machine in tilt. All the lights—or triggers—light up from a relatively slight jarring. These people are said to have a *secondary fibrositis*—secondary to underlying disk or facet joint strains. Fibrositis can also be seen in patients with low thyroid function, ankylosing spondylitis, polymyalgia rheumatica, viral infections (typically influenza), and after unaccustomed exercise or prolonged stressful posture—sleeping on the hard ground or on too soft a mattress. Some people, particularly middle-aged women, seem to develop a generalized fibrositis that has no apparent cause. It can wax and wane, worsen in cold damp weather, get better on vacation, and worsen with poor sleeping (and many patients have difficulty getting a restful sleep) and with emotional stress. These patients can be miserably uncomfortable, feel neurotic (since they are often told nothing is wrong, because no X-ray or blood test demonstrates any abnormality), and be concerned that they have a serious arthritis or worse. Treatment designed to relieve pain can include local massage, ice packs, ice massage, acupressure, and even acupuncture, as well as local anesthetic (Novocain or lidocaine) injections, sometimes mixed with small amounts of various forms of cortisone. These patients often benefit when their muscles are trained to relax, and this can be enhanced in some by the use of biofeedback and general relaxation exercises designed to take the tension out of muscles. Good diet, sleep restoration strategies, and general physical conditioning can help these patients maintain a normal lifestyle. Nonetheless, since symptoms wax and wane and are aggravated by emotional stress, psychological counseling and support groups (and in our Center, this can include simply talking to others with this disorder) can, in addition to the other treatments, help to keep the "safety" on the "triggers" and the symptoms from holding you up.

It is clear, then, that the ecology of our bodies is extremely well engineered and yet the conditions that can impact on our spine remain vulnerable to threats to our internal environment. Dis-ease, which means a lack of ease, or discomfort, or illness, can affect our backs due to ill advised use and abuse, or due to infectious and systemic disorders over which we have no control.

There are a variety of conditions that can affect the low back in a variety of manners, and with each category of symptoms there is often a wide range of intensity or severity of pain that accompanies the disorder. Since oftentimes we really don't know what it is that's causing our pain or discomfort, it's important to have a rational strategy for determining what might be wrong and what to do about it. Our assessment of the severity of our painful disorder is fundamental to our ability to take the proper steps to find out what's wrong and to ensure that we have the proper treatment. A few clouds in the sky may portend a forthcoming storm, or the passing of another lovely day. Dark clouds and thunderheads are a pretty good indicator that we're in for some stormy weather. We probably don't need a raincoat and umbrella when there are a few clouds in a sunny sky, but we might need raincoat, umbrella, and galloshes if the skies are lowering and raindrops have begun falling.

In Part II, we will learn how to determine whether we're in for fair weather or foul as far as our backs are concerned. We will learn how to determine the severity of our back pain problem and what decisions we should make in order to properly relieve it as expeditiously as possible.

II.

WHAT'S WRONG

WITH YOUR BACK

AND

HOW TO FIX IT

4.

THE

LOW BACK PAIN

DECISION TREE

Problem solving for back pain problems or any other problems is done in a systematic fashion, with the pros and cons of each issue given careful consideration before a decision is made. We speak of this step-by-step decision-making process as a "decision tree."

The decision tree is a very rational branching decision-making process that we all use, consciously or unconsciously, in our everyday lives. It is the basis for all computer functions. If you are driving on the highway to San Francisco and come to a branching of the road, you will read the signs and choose the road to San Francisco and not to Sacramento. If you go to a market for bread, you will select the bread counter out of all the food counters, and then you will select the kind of bread you want, the size, the freshness, and the price. Each of these decisions is made by comparing known choices and following the choice that best suits your particular needs. You are actually already climbing the decision tree. You have decided to back away from your low back pain. You purchased this book, you have read Part I, and you are now ready to make further intelligent choices.

The purpose of the decision tree for low back pain is to alert you to what is worth worrying about and to help you plan with your doctor the best approach to your treatment. Doctors are human and fallible. If your doctor has had a rough night or a very busy day, he just might overlook something he would ordinarily want to say or do for you—so ask him if he thinks this exercise or that corset or this test or treatment might be helpful; or, indeed, if you are concerned that any procedure might be harmful. Be sure you fully understand what you are to do and how you are to do it. Don't settle for "Take it easy," "Don't over-do," or "Be sure and get enough rest." You need to know how to tell *when* you are over-doing, and what *enough* means—one hour, two hours, eight hours in bed, on the couch, on a chair? You are the only one who has the ultimate control of the care for your back problems—so don't be embarrassed to ask about some of the suggestions on back protection or about the exercises that are presented in this book (*see Parts IV and V*).

Once you know where you are going and what you are after, you will get there more quickly, safely, and inexpensively by following a logical decision tree sequence. It does little good for your doctor to rush over and see an emergency if he has forgotten his medical bag, and it does equally little good to have expensive diagnostic tests performed or therapies and treatment provided if your problem is a simple one, e.g., morning back pain, and you've been sleeping on a lumpy mattress—get a new one (*see "The Mattress," pg. 177*).

The following several chapters are designed to help you and your doctor take the necessary steps to alleviate your low back pain problem.

5.

THE ROOT DECISION

AND

DANGER SIGNALS

The seed has been planted. The decision tree has taken root. You have made the root decision that you have a back pain problem and that you're going to do all that you can to get relief.

Good News for Bad Backs, the trunk of your decision tree, provides a sturdy support for the branching decision choices that you can make as you climb away from back pain.

DANGER SIGNALS

The first branch on your back pain decision tree may not support you. Check it out carefully for any Danger Signals. You've seen these before in Chapter 3.

If any of these danger signals are present, your decision is to take no risks and arrange to see your doctor directly, because these may be the signs and symptoms of arthritis, cancer, infection, or severe nerve pressure (*see Chapter 12, "What Kind of Doctor Should I See?"*).

With your feet firmly on the ground—or in your doctor's office—you can help your doctor decide what needs to be done

DANGER SIGNALS

1. Pain with no obvious cause
2. Pain gradual in onset and increasing in severity
3. Pain lasting more than three weeks
4. Pain and weakness or numbness in a leg
5. Pain unrelieved by rest, pain at night, pain for which there is no comfortable position
6. Pain and sickness, fever, chills, sweats, loss of appetite, nausea, weight loss
7. Pain and kidney or bladder dysfunction
8. Pain and constipation, diarrhea, or incontinence

next. He or she needs to know your medical history and background because there may be clues in your own past history or in that of your family that can help diagnose relatively uncommon, potentially serious problems. If your doctor asks about skin rash, eye inflammation, diarrhea, or swollen joints, he or she may be searching for clues that help diagnose ankylosing spondylitis, an arthritic type of spine disorder; or if he or she asks about dark urine stains on your underwear, he or she will be wondering if you have a rare metabolic condition called *ochronosis* that can cause a severe spinal arthritis.

DON'T BACK OFF

If your physician does not know you well, he or she may ask some very personal questions. Doctors need to know your state of mind—depression can cause or aggravate back pain and lead to loss of appetite, poor sleep, and sick feelings. Your doctor will want to know what your family is like, where you work, how you play, and how you pay your bills. You may say, "Anyone who hurts like I do is bound to feel depressed—just fix my back." But sometimes depression, triggered or aggravated by back pain, may be the major problem that requires treatment. It is well known that people who are significantly depressed respond poorly under treatment and in particular when operated on for back pain. For these patients, treatment of depression and treatment of the back must go hand-in-hand. It is interesting in light of this connection that small amounts of drugs used to treat depression are also useful in treating pain, even in non-depressed patients.

Your physician will want to know what medicines you have taken previously and, specifically, what narcotic or tranquilizing drugs, legally prescribed or otherwise purchased for so-called "recreational" drug use, you might be taking. Addiction to drugs used intravenously is associated with a high risk of infection, and patients who are addicted to narcotics for any reason ("recreational" stimulation or pain control) are notoriously difficult to treat until their drug problem is overcome.

Your doctor will want to know about any accidents you might have had, particularly if you have had an industrial accident or if you have a potential or actual lawsuit underway. It is unfortunate but true that a low back pain patient who does have a lawsuit or disability claim has about half the chance of getting well compared to one who does not. So don't be offended if your doctor gets personal. He or she doesn't know you as well as he might like and needs to know a lot about you to be able to effectively manage your low back problem.

THE DECISION TREE BEGINS BRANCHING IN YOUR OWN BACK YARD

So we've taken root, grown a trunk and a branch of your decision tree, and we've already begun pruning it. A variety of disorders on the first branch have been considered and eliminated in the pruning process including tumors, infection, arthritis, neuritis, muscle disease, and even blood vessel disease. In other words, you have a low back pain of the common garden variety with some disk deterioration and/or facet joint strain.

There are still many branches on your decision tree, even though the diagnosis seems now to be straightforward. The severity of your pain, the presence of sciatica, the duration of your symptoms, your general physical and psychological condition, and many other factors have to be considered so that you make the right decisions, climb out onto sturdy branches, and climb up and away from back pain.

6.

SELECTING

YOUR PAIN LEVEL:

THE MAJOR BRANCHING

DECISION

If you've got an acute or recurrent low back pain that has no serious disk overtones (paralysis or loss of bowel or bladder control) or other Danger Signals to worry about, there are still a number of things to think about and a number of decisions to make. Should you go to bed? If so, for how long? Should you wear a corset or a brace? If so, which one, and what kind? Should you take medicine, use traction, have manipulation, soak in a tub, use an ice pack, have ultrasound or transcutaneous nerve stimulation, have an injection, or what have you? First you must decide how severe your pain is. What is your *pain level?*

BACK HOME TREATMENT

No matter what your level of pain, you will have to consider the many treatment options appropriate to your problem and make the best possible choices to help relieve your pain and promote healing in your back. If your present pain level becomes less severe, you will want to choose those treatments, exercises, and activities that are appropriate for the new, improved level

TABLE 1	PAIN LEVELS AT A GLANCE	
PAIN	LEVEL	PAIN ACTIVITY CLUES
Severe	☀	Pain is very uncomfortable with any movement and at best you can only do minimal activity, e.g., get out of bed or sit and arise, and that with considerable discomfort or even almost intolerable pain.
Moderate	☼	Pain is very much there most of the time and definitely keeps you from vigorous or prolonged normal activity.
Mild	☼	Pain is there, especially noticeable with strains, overuse, or prolonged static posture such as bending, sitting, standing—it is rarely severe enough to stop you.
Minimal	○	Pain is usually not there, and if present, it does not interfere with your customary work and recreational activities.

that you have attained. Even if your pain is at a minimal level, you'll want to choose to keep it that way. It also won't hurt to know what to do if you over-do and the back pain starts back up* again.

Let's examine the many possibilities that need to be considered for you to select the safest and best treatments at home (Back Home Treatment) and what options you will want to be aware of when seeking professional medical care (Medical Back-Up).

BACK HOME TREATMENT

Back pain rarely chooses a convenient time or place to visit us. When it's severe enough to put us out of action or even to slow us down, we have to do something right away to get relief and to get going again, no matter where we are or how late the hour. We have to use Back Home Treatment.

There are two classes of Back Home Treatment: Back First Aid and Back Second Aid.

BACK HOME TREATMENT

BACK FIRST AID (R-I-C-E)
    Rest
    Ice
    Corset
    "Feel-Good" Easing Exercises

BACK SECOND AID
    Medicine Cabinet
    Back Rest and Protection (ergonomics)
    Home Therapy (heat, ice, traction)
    General Assistance
    Diet

■ *Back First Aid.* If your pain is now severe or has intensified, there are some very simple and straightforward things you can do to help relieve pain while waiting to see if you should check with your doctor. First of all, if in doubt, lie down on your back with your knees bent (*see Exercise #1, "Basic Pelvic Tilt," pg. 225*) and place an ice bag under or over the area that hurts. Leave it there for about 20 minutes out of every hour.

For a position of comfort in bed, place a firm pillow or a small suitcase or bolster under your knees to help maintain the bent knee and flat back posture. If side-lying is more comfortable, tighten your stomach and your buttocks (do a pelvic tilt) and roll like a log onto your side. Keep a small pillow between your knees for additional comfort. Some patients are actually more comfortable lying face-down. If this is the case, then it's probably okay for you. Lying face-down with a firm pillow under your stomach to take the arch out of your back may give you another position of comfort in bed.

If you must sit, select a firm chair with a supporting back. If you have an old corset or foundation garment that has helped you in the past, wear it. If there are exercises that consistently give you relief from pain, try them. We call this *Back First Aid*. First aid for backs is like first aid for any acute injury. The Red Cross mnemonic R-I-C-E (a fertile idea) stands for Rest (pelvic tilt position), Ice (cold pack), Compression (corset), and instead of Elevation, for Back First Aid we substitute "Feel-Good" Easing Exercises (*see Chapter 26*).

■ *Back Second Aid.* In addition to the First Aid measures, there are a number of additional choices that will help you relieve your back pain, enable you to function optimally, and expedite getting back into action. These are the *Back Second Aids*. They consist of: prescribed or over-the-counter pain-medications that you may have in your medicine chest or in your travel kit; protection techniques for dressing, grooming, sitting, standing, lying, packing, working, and pacing your activities to minimize back strain (*for more details on back protection, see Chapter 17*); therapies in addition to ice, such as heat, massage, and traction; assistive devices like a long-handled shoe horn, a reaching stick, or a cane; the employment of an assistant—housekeeper, nurse, chauffeur, or "gofer" (to *go for* this or that); and a nonconstipating, nourishing, and weight-stabilizing or weight-reduction diet.

One can't over-emphasize the value of using one's body efficiently and using appropriate tools and techniques in order to maximize that efficiency. In fact, a whole new science called *ergonomics* (*ergo* meaning work and *nomics* meaning economically) has emerged, and along with it, a variety of consultants to help individuals as well as industries function in a way that gets the maximum productivity with a minimum of disability.

MEDICAL BACK-UP

The more severe your back pain, the more urgent the need for medical consultation and supervision. If your back pain level is minimal and stays minimal, you may need professional advice only if you are considering a previously untried and potentially injurious activity, so that you can learn how to condition yourself properly to avoid back strain.

Medical Back-Up is essential for accurate diagnosis. Deciding whether you need special diagnostic or therapeutic procedures and possibly hospitalization obviously requires a physician. The duration of rest, the return to full- or part-time employment, the use of prescription drugs, corseting, specialized pain modalities, therapeutic exercises, manipulation, injections for pain control, acupuncture, physical therapy, occupational therapy, psychotherapy, or nursing—all require professional Medical Back-Up.

MEDICAL BACK-UP

OPTIONS

Medical Supervision and Hospital Care
Rest Prescribed
Medication Prescribed
Corset and Brace
Modalities Prescribed
Exercises Prescribed
Manipulation
Injections
Acupuncture
Health Care Assistance
Psychological and Social Counseling

After reviewing the major components of the decision tree, you are now ready to select your pain level. This major branching decision will determine the type of Back Home Treatment and Medical Back-Up you may need. Remember to refer back to this decision tree when your pain level has changed and has hopefully been reduced and your symptoms have eased.

SELECTING YOUR PAIN LEVEL—THE MAJOR BRANCHING DECISION

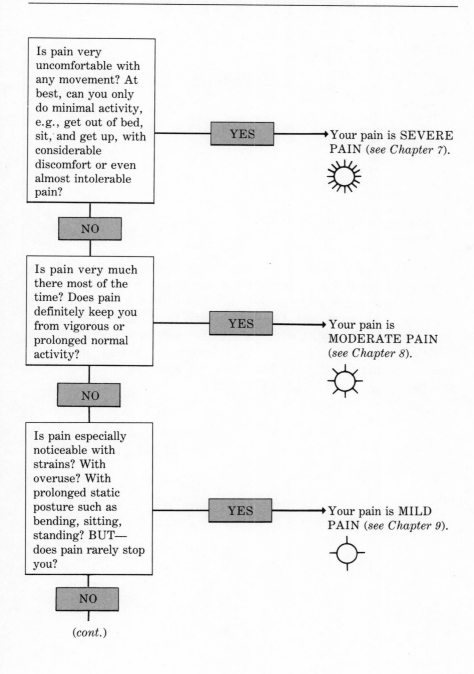

Is pain very uncomfortable with any movement? At best, can you only do minimal activity, e.g., get out of bed, sit, and get up, with considerable discomfort or even almost intolerable pain?

YES → Your pain is SEVERE PAIN (*see Chapter 7*).

NO

Is pain very much there most of the time? Does pain definitely keep you from vigorous or prolonged normal activity?

YES → Your pain is MODERATE PAIN (*see Chapter 8*).

NO

Is pain especially noticeable with strains? With overuse? With prolonged static posture such as bending, sitting, standing? BUT— does pain rarely stop you?

YES → Your pain is MILD PAIN (*see Chapter 9*).

NO

(*cont.*)

SELECTING YOUR PAIN LEVEL—THE MAJOR BRANCHING DECISION

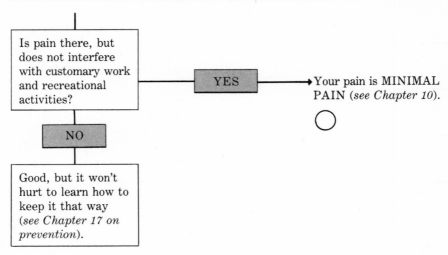

O.K. You've made your pain level decision and you know in general about Back Home Treatments and Medical Back-Up. So now you are ready to look up your pain level: Severe (4), Chapter 7; Moderate (3), Chapter 8; Mild (2), Chapter 9; Minimal (1), Chapter 10. Continue on the specific pain level branch of your decision tree and make the right decisions to help push your pain back down, get your back pain off your back, and get you and your back back in action.

7.

DECISIONS, DECISIONS,

DECISIONS FOR

SEVERE PAIN

If you have identified your pain as SEVERE, LEVEL 4, continue below on the SEVERE branch of your decision tree on page 50.

When back pain is severe, you can only think of how to get relief. Nothing else really matters. Back pain rarely comes on at a convenient time. Fortunately, the key elements of Back First Aid (Rest, Ice, Corset, and "Feel-Good" Easing Exercises) are usually at hand or readily available. Back Second Aid includes household medications and simple measures to help you minimize back pain while getting through the unavoidable activities of the day. Back Second Aids provide the basics for containing severe back pain until professional Medical Back-Up for proper diagnosis and medically supervised treatment is obtained.

DECISION TREE—☼

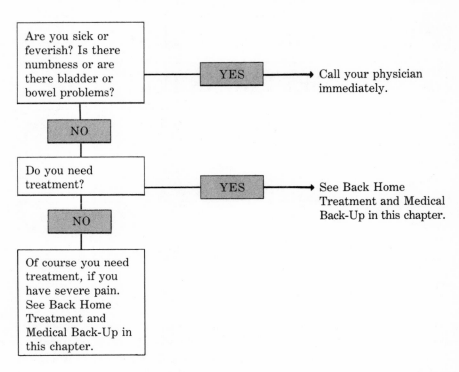

Are you sick or feverish? Is there numbness or are there bladder or bowel problems?

YES → Call your physician immediately.

NO

Do you need treatment?

YES → See Back Home Treatment and Medical Back-Up in this chapter.

NO

Of course you need treatment, if you have severe pain. See Back Home Treatment and Medical Back-Up in this chapter.

BACK HOME TREATMENT—SEVERE PAIN

BACK FIRST AID

REST

This is Back in Bed for bedrest time! Bedrest for severe pain means 90% or more of the day is spent in bed. Sex should be on the back burner—abstain! Carefully review techniques for getting in and out of bed, brushing your teeth, and getting on or off the floor (*see Back Protection Principles in Chapter 17*). When your pain level is severe, your only outing is to see the doctor.

ICE

Cold packs applied over or under the painful areas for 20 minutes as often as every hour may help reduce severe pain. If you do not tolerate the cold packs, but find heat soothing, it's okay to use heat for 20 minutes out of each hour. Avoid soaking in a warm tub—climbing back out can be hazardous.

CORSETS
AND
BRACES

If you've worn a corset for the same problem before and it still fits comfortably, wear it in bed if it helps, and whenever you have to get up out of bed.

EASING
EXERCISES

Stop all previous exercises. Cautiously try "Feel-Good" Easing Exercises (*see Chapter 26*) and repeat any or all of these exercises (if they do not increase pain) three times, gently, every hour or two.

BACK FIRST AID DECISION CHECK LIST ☼

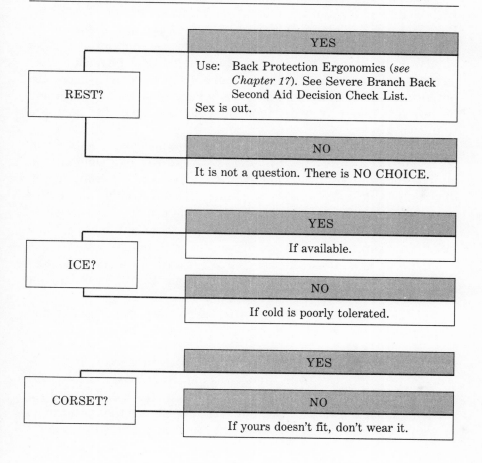

REST?

YES

Use: Back Protection Ergonomics (*see Chapter 17*). See Severe Branch Back Second Aid Decision Check List.
Sex is out.

NO

It is not a question. There is NO CHOICE.

ICE?

YES

If available.

NO

If cold is poorly tolerated.

CORSET?

YES

NO

If yours doesn't fit, don't wear it.

BACK FIRST AID DECISION CHECK LIST ☼

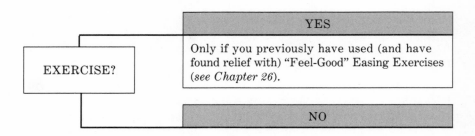

	YES
EXERCISE?	Only if you previously have used (and have found relief with) "Feel-Good" Easing Exercises (*see Chapter 26*).
	NO

BACK SECOND AID

- *Medication.*

  Narcotics—Narcotic tablets you may have on hand: Aspirin with Codeine, Tylenol with Codeine, Vicodin, Darvon, Darvocet, Percocet, and Talwin. *Check with a physician before self-medicating.* These drugs can cause severe constipation, so drink plenty of fluids and eat a high fiber diet. Your physician may suggest the use of laxatives or stool softeners. These drugs are potentially habit-forming, but there is very little risk of addiction if they are taken as prescribed by your physician for no more than two weeks.

  Nonnarcotic analgesics (pain relievers) and nonsteroidal (non-cortisone) anti-inflammatory drugs—Anaprox and Dolobid are equivalent to two to three aspirin tablets or acetaminophen (Tylenol) tablets and rarely are adequate for control of severe pain. Nonsteroidal anti-inflammatory drugs are also equivalent to aspirin and Tylenol for controlling or, more often, not very effectively controlling most really *severe* back pain.

  Muscle relaxers—Robaxin, Soma, Flexeril, Parafon, or Valium may help sedate you because they are primarily tranquilizers, but otherwise do little for severe pain.

  OTC (over-the-counter) remedies—See "Over-the-Counter and Through the Woods" in Chapter 15.

- *Back Protection Ergonomics.* Learn Back Protection Principle #2, "Down and Up from Bed" (*see pg. 151*), Back Protection Principle #1, the "Four Back Words" (*see pg. 148*), and Back Protection Principle #4, "Hip Bending" (*see pg. 155*) so that you can go forward, getting through the day with the least possible discomfort!

■ *General Assistance.* Get all the help you need for everything—from bathing and meal preparation to business.

■ *Diet.* Pain medication and inactivity can upset your digestive system. Note these daily features:

Bland—Avoid gassy or exotic foods.

Fluids—Drink the equivalent of eight glasses of fluids; substitute no more than two glasses of wine or beer (taken with food).

Fiber—Eat a high-fiber diet, with foods such as bran and salads to provide bulk, especially if you are taking constipating drugs.

Calories—2000 calories a day should be enough when you're resting.

Vitamins—No additional vitamins are needed.

Calcium Supplements—Not helpful for severe pain level.

BACK SECOND AID DECISION CHECK LIST ☼

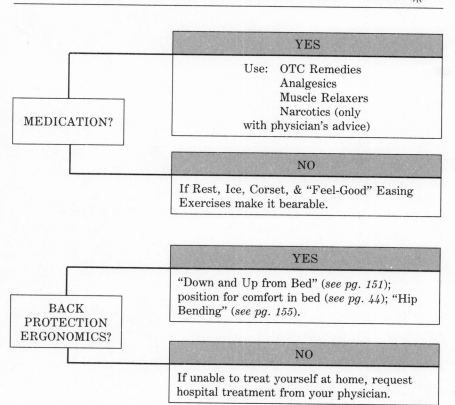

MEDICATION?	**YES**
	Use: OTC Remedies Analgesics Muscle Relaxers Narcotics (only with physician's advice)
	NO
	If Rest, Ice, Corset, & "Feel-Good" Easing Exercises make it bearable.

BACK PROTECTION ERGONOMICS?	**YES**
	"Down and Up from Bed" (*see pg. 151*); position for comfort in bed (*see pg. 44*); "Hip Bending" (*see pg. 155*).
	NO
	If unable to treat yourself at home, request hospital treatment from your physician.

BACK SECOND AID DECISION CHECK LIST ☼

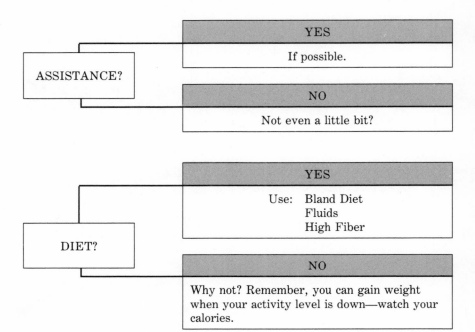

ASSISTANCE?	YES
	If possible.

	NO
	Not even a little bit?

DIET?	YES
	Use: Bland Diet
	Fluids
	High Fiber

	NO
	Why not? Remember, you can gain weight when your activity level is down—watch your calories.

MEDICAL BACK-UP—SEVERE PAIN ☼

First and foremost is the doctor's *correct diagnosis.*

■ *Hospitalization.* Your physician may decide that hospitalization could be necessary for pain control, diagnosis, and specialized treatments.

■ *Rest*—Obviously, rest is essential.

■ *Medications (Supervised)*—Oral and occasionally injectable narcotics may be prescribed. High-dose steroids are used on occasion for severe, unrelenting back pain. If you are taking Back Second Aid medications, check with your physician regarding how much of which medicine and how long to take it. Your home remedies may not be compatible with prescribed medications.

- *Corset* (Prescription). Your doctor may prescribe a quickly fitted, easily adjusted elastic corset as a temporary measure.

- *Modalities.*

  TNS (Transcutaneous Nerve Stimulation)—Particularly for sciatic pain, can be applied by a therapist when prescribed. Can be used as a home pain control treatment with proper patient and/or family instruction. There are few side effects, other than from electrode irritation.

  Traction—Potentially dangerous in patients with sciatica, it is best avoided at least for the first 2–4 days after the onset of severe symptoms associated with sciatic pain.

  Massage—Avoid except over unrelated areas such as the neck or arm.

- *Exercise*—As prescribed.

- *Manipulation*—Potentially dangerous and best to avoid, particularly if sciatic nerve irritation is present.

- *Injections.*

  Narcotic—morphine or Demerol intramuscularly may be required on rare occasion for very severe pain.

  "Trigger or tender point" injections—Injections of a local anesthetic into a tender area of muscle attachment or muscle spasm may bring about prompt relief that can sometimes last for hours or days. The anesthetic is often combined with a small amount of a cortisone or "steroid" type drug.

  Facet joint injections—Injection of a cortisone-steroid drug into irritated facet joints is sometimes useful to relieve severe pain.

  Epidural blocks—Injections of a cortisone-steroid drug into the epidural space (a fatty layer that surrounds the spinal cord) at a place where a painful disk or irritated spinal nerve emerges. These are often helpful in controlling pain and sciatica.

- *Acupuncture.* Can help relieve even severe pain, at least temporarily, in some patients.

- *Health Care Assistance.* Ask about the Visiting Nurse Association, Home Health Care agencies or homemaker assistance for home therapy and assistance in meeting your daily needs.

■ *Psychological, Social, and Medical Counseling.* These may be required to help you through a stressful period and to deal with any complications that might arise.

MEDICAL BACK-UP OPTIONS

You'll want to consider the following questions when you see your physician and other health professionals because of severe back pain. (*More detailed information on these topics is included in Chapter 12.*)

TABLE 2   MEDICAL BACK-UP OPTIONS—☼

		COMMENTS		
		USUALLY HELPFUL	SOMETIMES HELPFUL	POTENTIALLY DANGEROUS
Hospital	If arrangements for home treatments are not feasible			
Rest		X		
Medications		X		
Corset or brace		X		
Modalities for pain				
Heat			X	
Cold		X		
Massage				X
Traction			X	X
TNS (transcutaneous nerve stimulation)			X	
Exercise			X	X
Manipulation				with sciatica

TABLE 2   MEDICAL BACK-UP OPTIONS—☼

	COMMENTS		
	USUALLY HELPFUL	SOMETIMES HELPFUL	POTENTIALLY DANGEROUS
Injections			
Narcotic	X		X
Trigger points	X		
Facet Joint		X	
Epidural	X		X
Acupuncture		X	
Health Care Assistance	X		
Psychological/Social/Medical Counseling	X		

MEDICAL BACK-UP DECISION CHECK LIST—☼

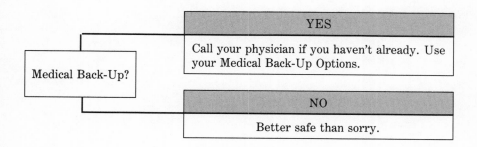

	YES
	Call your physician if you haven't already. Use your Medical Back-Up Options.
Medical Back-Up?	
	NO
	Better safe than sorry.

CONCLUSION

If your pain level is SEVERE, you're going to need to rest. If you're going to rest, you need to know how to get in and out of bed or in and out of a chair, and how to take care of your minimum daily needs. You probably will need some medicine. You should certainly consult your physician, and you may find that cold applications and a corset can help relieve your discomfort.

But severe pain rarely lasts for more than a few days, and when it moderates somewhat, you may have to make decisions for a more moderate pain level. Let's move on then to the next chapters to find out how to deal with the conditions that we may face as the pain lessens in intensity. Your back pain problem is mending, but is not yet mended. Many opportunities will now present themselves to help you get through the periods of time when your back pain is still a problem but, fortunately, is not as severe as it started out to be. In Chapter 8 we will learn how to deal with a moderate pain level.

8.

DECISIONS,

DECISIONS FOR

MODERATE PAIN

You have identified your pain level as MODERATE. If you have improved from a severe pain level or if your pain level has never been more than moderate, you should now proceed on the MODERATE PAIN, LEVEL 3 branch of your decision tree. It still may be useful to take a backward glance at the Severe Pain, Level 4 Back Home Treatments. There may be some Back First Aid or Back Second Aid suggestions that can come in handy even though you're looking forward to getting back out.

DECISION TREE—☼

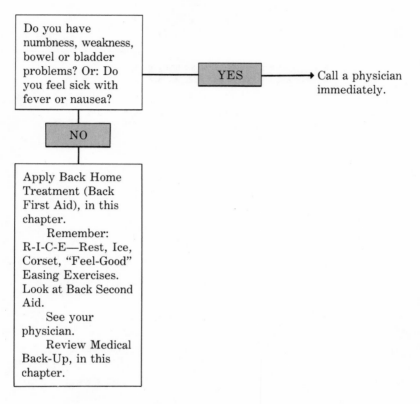

Do you have numbness, weakness, bowel or bladder problems? Or: Do you feel sick with fever or nausea?

YES → Call a physician immediately.

NO

Apply Back Home Treatment (Back First Aid), in this chapter.
    Remember: R-I-C-E—Rest, Ice, Corset, "Feel-Good" Easing Exercises.
Look at Back Second Aid.
    See your physician.
    Review Medical Back-Up, in this chapter.

BACK HOME TREATMENT—MODERATE PAIN ☼

BACK FIRST AID

REST   Initially you should be up only to go to the bathroom, for meals and other essentials, and for doctor visits. With improvement, increase "up" time progressively from 10% to 90% of the day. Rest is an "active" and often the most difficult part of your treatment when you reach the stage in your recovery when you can be up and around.

Rest without guilt. Rest is part of your treatment program because it relieves pain, promotes healing, and allows you to make progress on your back-reconditioning exercise program. When you are resting or napping, you are "actively" treating your back and not lying down on the job. If you're feeling up to it, check out Chapter 23, "Back in Love."

ICE

Use a cold pack for 15 to 20 minutes every hour if needed, or at least four times a day over the painful area. Wrap an ice bag (cold pack or a pack of frozen peas) in a warm, moist hand towel, and apply over or under (whatever is easiest) the painful area (back, buttock, or leg). The warm towel minimizes the initial chilling discomfort. Ice massage, with water frozen in a Dixie cup, for 2 to 3 minutes can relieve painful sore spots.

Hot packs can be helpful for patients who do not tolerate cold.

CORSETS AND BRACES

You'll probably need one to get up and about with any comfort. You may even find it helpful when lying in bed. Be sure the prescribed corset fits and that you can get in and out of it easily.

EASING EXERCISES

Stay with the "Feel-Good" Easing Exercises in Chapter 26 that are comfortable. You can try the Knee Back (Lying and Sitting) exercises, which may provide additional comfort (*see pp. 235, 236*).

BACK FIRST AID DECISION CHECK LIST—☼

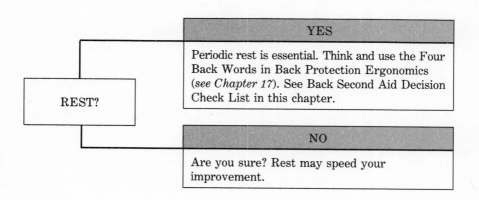

	YES
REST?	Periodic rest is essential. Think and use the Four Back Words in Back Protection Ergonomics (*see Chapter 17*). See Back Second Aid Decision Check List in this chapter.
	NO
	Are you sure? Rest may speed your improvement.

BACK FIRST AID DECISION CHECK LIST–☼

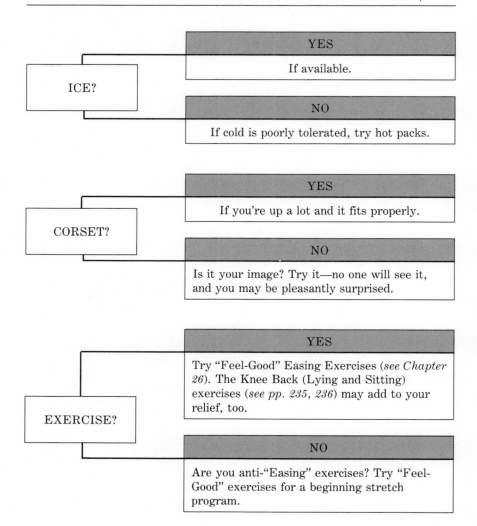

ICE?	
YES	If available.
NO	If cold is poorly tolerated, try hot packs.

CORSET?	
YES	If you're up a lot and it fits properly.
NO	Is it your image? Try it—no one will see it, and you may be pleasantly surprised.

EXERCISE?	
YES	Try "Feel-Good" Easing Exercises (*see Chapter 26*). The Knee Back (Lying and Sitting) exercises (*see pp. 235, 236*) may add to your relief, too.
NO	Are you anti-"Easing" exercises? Try "Feel-Good" exercises for a beginning stretch program.

BACK SECOND AID

■ *Rest.* See Back Second Aid Decision Check List, in this chapter.

■ *Back Protection Ergonomics.* You are gradually getting up and around more. You can't be too careful! Do what you have to do (work = *ergo*) as efficiently (eco-nomically) as possible. Let the

Four Back Words be the passwords to a pain-free back. BACK FIRST: plan ahead to spare your back. BACK FLAT: tighten your stomach and squeeze your buttocks before initiating any new movement or activity. BACK STRAIGHT: avoid bending, twisting, and reaching. BACK LAST: use your arms, legs, ladders, or reaching tools first, and your back will last! Plan thoughtfully for both quiet and active times. You might be pleasantly surprised at how much easier it is to get around with a cane for awhile. Try it—you might like it. You can always walk away from it if you don't. If your back pain is moderate, the same principles for severe back pain still apply. You want to do all that you can to minimize unnecessary pain. Think and act ergonomically. Don't waste pain!

FOUR BACK WORDS

BACK FIRST
BACK FLAT
BACK STRAIGHT
BACK LAST

■ *General Assistance.* Use your head—not your *back*. You probably need help for some chores, such as housework, driving, shopping, and travel. A tip to the porter while traveling is an investment in preventive medicine. If you need help and it's painful to ask, remember, it may be more painful if you don't!

■ *Diet.* Keep it digestible, low caloric, and nonconstipating.

■ *Medications.* See Back Second Aid Decision Check List on pg. 64.

■ *Home Therapies.* See Back Second Aid Decision Check List on pg. 64.

■ *Exercise.* See Back Second Aid Decision Check List on pg. 64.

BACK SECOND AID DECISION CHECK LIST—☼

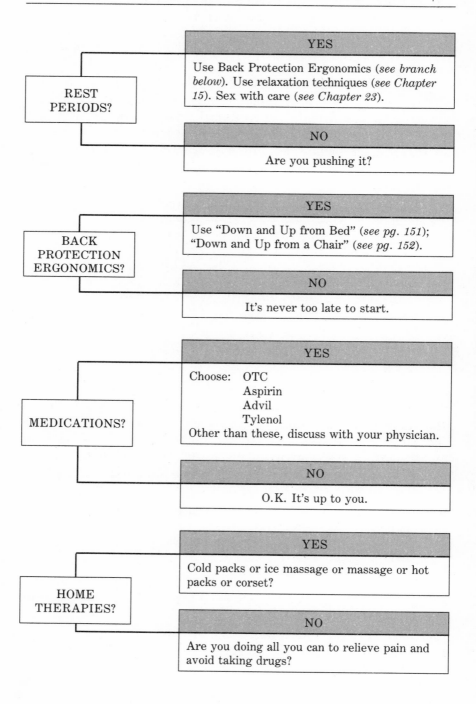

REST PERIODS?

YES

Use Back Protection Ergonomics (*see branch below*). Use relaxation techniques (*see Chapter 15*). Sex with care (*see Chapter 23*).

NO

Are you pushing it?

BACK PROTECTION ERGONOMICS?

YES

Use "Down and Up from Bed" (*see pg. 151*); "Down and Up from a Chair" (*see pg. 152*).

NO

It's never too late to start.

MEDICATIONS?

YES

Choose: OTC
          Aspirin
          Advil
          Tylenol
Other than these, discuss with your physician.

NO

O.K. It's up to you.

HOME THERAPIES?

YES

Cold packs or ice massage or massage or hot packs or corset?

NO

Are you doing all you can to relieve pain and avoid taking drugs?

BACK SECOND AID DECISION CHECK LIST—☼

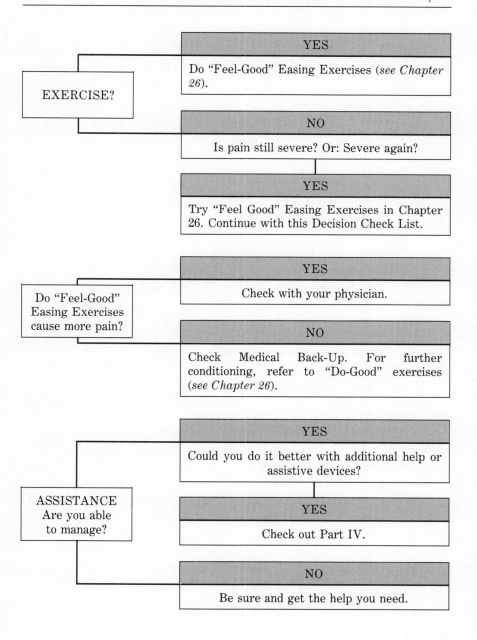

EXERCISE?

YES

Do "Feel-Good" Easing Exercises (*see Chapter 26*).

NO

Is pain still severe? Or: Severe again?

YES

Try "Feel Good" Easing Exercises in Chapter 26. Continue with this Decision Check List.

Do "Feel-Good" Easing Exercises cause more pain?

YES

Check with your physician.

NO

Check Medical Back-Up. For further conditioning, refer to "Do-Good" exercises (*see Chapter 26*).

ASSISTANCE Are you able to manage?

YES

Could you do it better with additional help or assistive devices?

YES

Check out Part IV.

NO

Be sure and get the help you need.

BACK SECOND AID DECISION CHECK LIST—☼

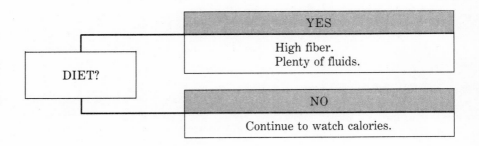

DIET?	YES
	High fiber. Plenty of fluids.
	NO
	Continue to watch calories.

MEDICAL BACK-UP—MODERATE PAIN 3

■ *Hospitalization.* Rarely necessary at this stage.

■ *Rest.* Check with your doctor as to when to increase your activity level and by how much.

■ *Medications.* Avoid pain by proper back protective ergonomics —do not use medication to mask pain except for urgent matters. Unlike aspirin, ibuprofen (Advil), and acetaminophen (Tylenol), the following medicines require prescriptions:

Narcotics—Narcotic tablets should be used sparingly. Check with a physician before self-medicating.

Nonnarcotic analgesics (pain relievers)—Nonnarcotic analgesics (pain relievers) and nonsteroidal (non-cortisone) anti-inflammatory drugs may be helpful in taking the edge off of your moderate pain level.

Muscle relaxers—These, too, will occasionally help take the edge off your pain, but rarely are necessary for more than a week or two.

Tranquilizers—A number of these drugs cause sedation and muscle spasm relaxation. Valium is probably the most popular. All tranquilizers are potentially habit-forming, interfere with thinking, and are not to be used if one is driving.

■ *Corset or Brace.* This should be carefully prescribed and fitted. Don't accept a corset or brace until you are sure that you know exactly how to don and doff it without aggravating your back. Ask when it's time to cut back on wearing your appliance. The goal is to get rid of it if possible, or to wear it only for vigorous or stressful activities.

■ *Modalities for Pain.*

TNS (transcutaneous nerve stimulation)—can often relieve back pain, particularly sciatic pain. Aside from electrode irritation, there are few side effects, and with proper instruction TNS can be used at home.

Traction—This can be helpful. Simple home units are available for rent or purchase, and they can easily be used in bed or on the floor. Some people find hanging from a door, in a sling, or upside-down helpful. (*Before considering traction, see Chapter 15.*)

Spray and stretch—This can be a cool way to relieve painful muscle spasm (*see Chapter 15*).

Massage—Skilled professional massage or acupressure (shiatsu) can help give temporary pain relief (*see Chapter 15*).

■ *Exercise*—As your pain eases, you should be instructed by your health professional in your "Do-Good" reconditioning exercises (*see Chapter 26*). These exercises should progress in harmony with your recovery. Abdominal strengthening exercises can keep your stomach firm, even while you are still wearing a corset.

■ *Manipulation*—Manipulation for a moderately painful lower back of a few days duration, due to disk or facet joint strains (particularly in the absence of sciatic nerve root compression) is relatively safe and may be effective in relieving pain. One to two manipulations per week for a maximum of four weeks should give the full measure of any benefit to be derived. If manipulation is used, it should be considered as part of the total treatment program—exercise, back protection ergonomics, therapy modalities, medication—and not as the treatment per se.

■ *Injections.* The use of relatively simple and safe local trigger point injections can often play an important role on the road *back* from back pain. Less often, the more difficult and more risky epidural steroid or facet joint injections can help turn the tide.

■ *Acupuncture.* Acupuncture is poorly understood, but nonetheless has a role as a safe pain-control therapy. It is relatively expensive and it does not work for everyone, but in some patients it is helpful and worth a try.

■ *Psychological, Social, and Medical Counseling.* If pain and disability are creating emotional stress, seek psychological counseling. If financial and family problems are getting out of hand, seek social counseling. Sex is permissible, but needs some planning (*see Chapter 23, "Back in Love"*).

MEDICAL BACK-UP OPTIONS

Use Medical Back-Up Options to help you prepare questions for your visit to your physician and other health professionals because of moderate back pain. (*See additional information on these topics in Chapter 12*).

TABLE 3 MEDICAL BACK-UP OPTIONS—☼

		USUALLY HELPFUL	SOMETIMES HELPFUL	POTENTIALLY DANGEROUS
Hospital	If arrangements for home treatment are not feasible			
Rest		X		
Medications		X		
Corset or brace		X		
Modalities for pain				
Heat		X		
Cold		X		
Massage			X	
Traction			X	X
TNS (transcutaneous nerve stimulation)			X	

TABLE 3 MEDICAL BACK-UP OPTIONS— ☼

| | | COMMENTS | |
	USUALLY HELPFUL	SOMETIMES HELPFUL	POTENTIALLY DANGEROUS
Exercise	X		X
Manipulation		X	with sciatica
Injections			
Narcotic		X	X
Trigger points	X		
Facet Joint		X	
Epidural		X	X
Acupuncture		X	
Health Care Assistance	X		
Psychological/Social/Medical Counseling		X	

MEDICAL BACK-UP DECISION CHECK LIST— ☼

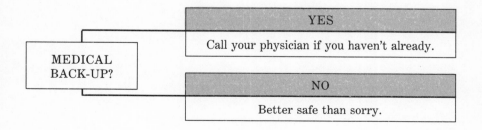

MEDICAL BACK-UP?	YES
	Call your physician if you haven't already.
	NO
	Better safe than sorry.

CONCLUSION

When your back pain level is MODERATE it's imperative that you have an accurate diagnosis and that you learn to do what you must do in a manner that minimizes unnecessary back stress and strain. Rest will help promote healing, and exercise can be useful both to help relieve the pain (*see "Feel-Good" Easing Exercises in Chapter 26*) and to begin a gradual reconditioning process (*see "Do-Good" exercises in Chapter 26*). Use medication as necessary, but only as necessary. Be patient with your back now, so that you can become an ex-back-pain-patient in the future. If you've followed the advice in this chapter, you are probably about ready to get on with the healing process and move to a mild pain level. Chapter 9 will help you through that period as expeditiously as possible.

9.

DECISIONS

FOR

MILD PAIN

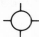

In the final analysis, pain is exactly what you say it is. No one can experience it for you and no one can put it into words for you. Progress in pain research has been extremely slow because there is no generally agreed upon way to measure the intensity of pain, let alone its meaning, for any given individual. One thing is clear: Pain that can be induced in the laboratory is experienced differently from pain that occurs due to bodily injury or illness. Nonetheless, we all, through the various and sundry traumas of life, come to know what severe, moderate, and mild pain is for us. You and you alone can make the determination of whether or not your back pain is mild. Don't make the mistake, as so many of us do, of denying that you have a back pain problem. It's important that you recognize that the pain is there and categorize it appropriately according to its pain level. That way, you can deal with it, make the right decisions, and get your back pain well behind you.

So your back pain is MILD. If it was severe, or even moderate, then mild is a blessing. But it could get worse, and happily, it could get better. If your back pain has never been more than mild, you will be well served to learn how to continue to protect your back by avoiding back strain and by properly conditioning your muscles. If you're not now doing back conditioning exercises, you'll benefit from a conditioning program beginning with Severe Pain, Level 4 exercises and progressing through to at least the Mild Pain, Level 2 exercises (*see Chapter 26*). When you have properly conditioned yourself, you can plan to enjoy a number of more vigorous athletic activities, such as swimming, cycling, walking, and for those with more exotic tastes, even yoga.

Now let's look at your options on the decision tree. First let's be sure that we have selected the correct branch, the MILD PAIN, LEVEL 2 branch, because there are a lot of good choices to be made, and you want to be sure that you're making the right ones.

DECISION TREE—◇-

Are you sure your pain is MILD?	**YES** →	See Back Home Treatment (First and Second Aid); Medical Back-Up; Back to Sports, in this chapter.
NO ↓		
Is your back pain MINIMAL PAIN?	**YES** →	Go on to next chapter, MINIMAL PAIN.
NO ↓		
Is it usually MILD PAIN, but presently MODERATE PAIN, or SEVERE PAIN? Is it back again?	**YES** →	Go back to MODERATE PAIN (*see Chapter 8*) until you're again ready for MILD PAIN.
NO ↓		
Check your pain level again (*see Table 1, page 43*).		

BACK HOME TREATMENT—MILD PAIN 2

By and large, when you're at a mild pain level, the thrust of your treatment is self-care and prevention. You'll want to be sure and do your exercises at least once, and preferably twice, daily; use your body as ergonomically as possible; and use medication as sparingly as possible. You'll want to be sure you're stretched out and limbered up before taking exercise or attempting more vigorous activity than usual, and always keep a little energy in reserve. Sometimes, despite your best intentions, the back pain of Level 2 will rear its ugly head. Then it's time to make the right decisions for Back Home Treatment for Mild Pain, Level 2.

BACK HOME TREATMENT DECISION TREE

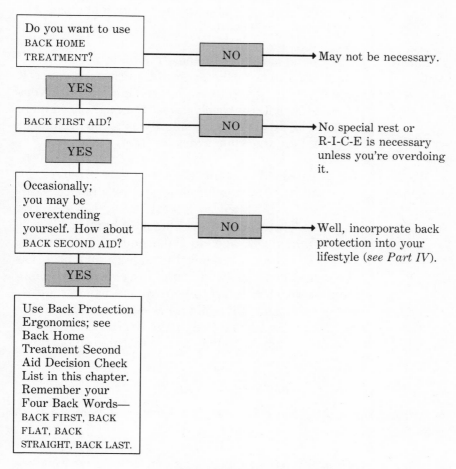

Do you want to use BACK HOME TREATMENT?

NO → May not be necessary.

YES

BACK FIRST AID?

NO → No special rest or R-I-C-E is necessary unless you're overdoing it.

YES

Occasionally; you may be overextending yourself. How about BACK SECOND AID?

NO → Well, incorporate back protection into your lifestyle (see Part IV).

YES

Use Back Protection Ergonomics; see Back Home Treatment Second Aid Decision Check List in this chapter. Remember your Four Back Words— BACK FIRST, BACK FLAT, BACK STRAIGHT, BACK LAST.

BACK FIRST AID

REST   You can be up and about without special rest unless you're overtired or engaged in unusual exertion.

Pace yourself so that you always have some energy stored up in reserve. Sex is now a matter of your personal comfort and pleasure.

ICE   Ice is nice when you need it, especially an ice massage over persistent sore spots for 2 to 3 minutes. Freeze water in a paper cup to make a handy massager. You can't go too far wrong with a cold pack. Wrap an ice bag (cold pack or a pack of frozen peas) in a warm moist hand towel, and apply over or under the painful area. (The warm towel minimizes the initial chilling discomfort.)

CORSETS   You should rarely need one. If you do, use the least
AND   supportive previously prescribed brace, and use it
BRACES   only if you are going to be engaged in unusual or very vigorous activities, when you feel you might need more protection. It will serve primarily as a good reminder wrapped around your waist to "keep you in line."

EASING   Do "Feel-Good" Easing Exercises (*see Chapter 26*)
EXERCISES   for comfort. For conditioning and preventive exer-
(DURING A   cises, go back down to Severe Pain, Level 4 and
FLARE-UP)   then Moderate Pain, Level 3 conditioning exercises (*see Chapter 26*), and do them gently, twice daily. Increase exercise intensity gradually and progress through all of the Mild Pain, Level 2 conditioning exercises and back up to your maintenance routine. Follow with the "Five-Minute Back Saver" (*see Chapter 28*). Listen to your body—the voices talking behind your back may be telling you something important.

BACK SECOND AID

■ *Medications.* See Back Second Aid Decision Check List, in this chapter.

■ *Back Protection Ergonomics.* Pace yourself, listen to your body— especially if you are getting *back* talk. Remember, BACK FIRST, BACK FLAT, BACK STRAIGHT, BACK LAST.

     Don't "waste pain"—Be sure that you have a supporting

mattress, a proper seat, and use good body mechanics at home, at work, and when traveling (*see Part IV*).

Take a Back Seat—Use a chair with good support, and add a towel or pillow that supports you properly (*see Chapter 18*).

Don't sit on the money—If you carry a wallet in your hip pocket, don't sit on it. It may cause the spine to tilt and add to your back strain.

Look at your shoes—An upright fellow needs a firm *understanding*: Wear supporting shoes. If you have knocked knees, flat feet, or a short leg, have shoe corrections made to support your feet properly. An upright gal has her feet on the ground: no heel over 1¼ inches. Check all your recreational footgear for proper fit and well cushioned soles.

Your work environment—be sure it is, insofar as possible, modified to minimize back stress (*see Chapter 24*).

Strategic withdrawal from pain—If repeated activity or prolonged activity is beginning to get you in the back, back off, do something else, do your back protective "Feel-Good" Easing Exercises in Chapter 26. It is better to finish the project a little later in the day than to spend tomorrow in bed with back pain.

■ *Rest Periods.* See Back Second Aid Decision Check List, below.

■ *General Assistance.* See Back Second Aid Decision Check List on pg. 76.

■ *Diet.* See Back Second Aid Decision Check List on pg. 76.

■ *Exercise.* The Back "Vitamin" is your daily exercise maintenance program. You should spend 10 to 20 minutes total per day on your back exercises, and do them at least once daily. Be consistent about your daily exercise program, because jumping into sporadic therapeutic or recreational exercise for which you are not properly conditioned can do more harm than good.

Be S-A-F-E. Be **S**trong enough, **A**gile enough, **F**lexible enough, and have enough **E**ndurance to engage in the contemplated exercise activity. Do a warm-up before and a cool-down after each recreational exercise section (*see "Warm-Up, Cool-Down," pg. 277*).

Back Bends Standing (*see Exercise #6, pg. 234*)—If you've found this comfortable and easy to do (*see "Feel-Good" Easing Exercises in Chapter 26*), repeat 5 to 10 times before and after unusual static (a long movie or concert; an automobile, plane, or bike ride) or active physical activities.

S   Be STRONG enough
A   AGILE enough
F   FLEXIBLE enough
E   have enough ENDURANCE
    for exercise activities

BACK SECOND AID DECISION CHECK LIST ✣

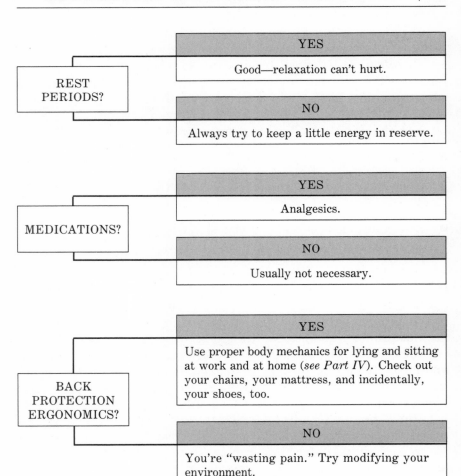

REST PERIODS?	YES
	Good—relaxation can't hurt.
	NO
	Always try to keep a little energy in reserve.

MEDICATIONS?	YES
	Analgesics.
	NO
	Usually not necessary.

BACK PROTECTION ERGONOMICS?	YES
	Use proper body mechanics for lying and sitting at work and at home (*see Part IV*). Check out your chairs, your mattress, and incidentally, your shoes, too.
	NO
	You're "wasting pain." Try modifying your environment.

BACK SECOND AID DECISION CHECK LIST ⬦

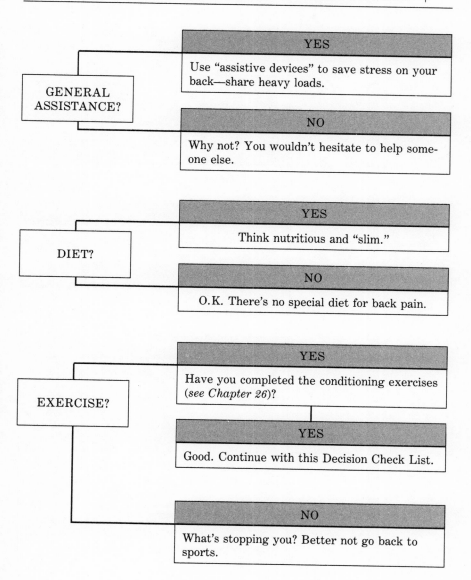

GENERAL ASSISTANCE?

YES

Use "assistive devices" to save stress on your back—share heavy loads.

NO

Why not? You wouldn't hesitate to help someone else.

DIET?

YES

Think nutritious and "slim."

NO

O.K. There's no special diet for back pain.

EXERCISE?

YES

Have you completed the conditioning exercises (*see Chapter 26*)?

YES

Good. Continue with this Decision Check List.

NO

What's stopping you? Better not go back to sports.

BACK SECOND AID DECISION CHECK LIST ✛

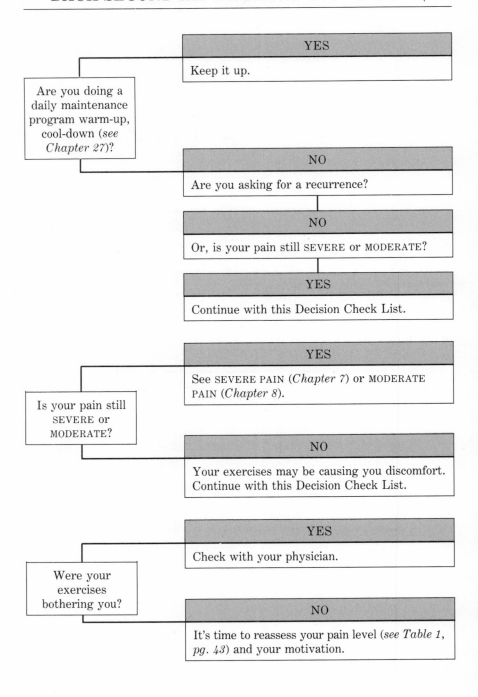

Are you doing a daily maintenance program warm-up, cool-down (*see Chapter 27*)?

YES
Keep it up.

NO
Are you asking for a recurrence?

NO
Or, is your pain still SEVERE or MODERATE?

YES
Continue with this Decision Check List.

Is your pain still SEVERE or MODERATE?

YES
See SEVERE PAIN (*Chapter 7*) or MODERATE PAIN (*Chapter 8*).

NO
Your exercises may be causing you discomfort. Continue with this Decision Check List.

Were your exercises bothering you?

YES
Check with your physician.

NO
It's time to reassess your pain level (*see Table 1, pg. 43*) and your motivation.

BACK TO SPORTS

These are the best all-around sports choices for recovering back pain patients (*see also Chapter 29, "Back to Sports"*):

■ *Swimming*—if you are a competent swimmer, is great. If not, take lessons and/or try a floatation belt—no diving, and avoid butterfly, breast stroke, and arching your neck and back.

■ *Cycling*—It's a good idea to start on an Exercycle with no resistance. Sit upright and keep the seat low enough to avoid twisting your pelvis (and back) when pedaling. Once you're in shape, bending over racing handlebars may be okay.

■ *Walking*—vigorously, in good shoes, over level, preferably soft turf.

■ *Race walking*—is probably more stressful than jogging. Avoid both, but if you can tolerate jogging and must *jog*, stay on soft, level turf and *walk* downhill. Try a treadmill for less jolt to the back.

■ *Yoga*—this takes supervision, patience, and training, and when the most exotic maneuvers, such as headstands, are eliminated, yoga can be a useful, relaxing, stretching and strengthening regimen.

BACK TO SPORTS DECISION CHECK LIST—◇

BACK TO SPORTS?	YES
	Good. Continue with this Decision Check List.
	NO
	Reconsider.

BACK TO SPORTS DECISION CHECK LIST—⌀

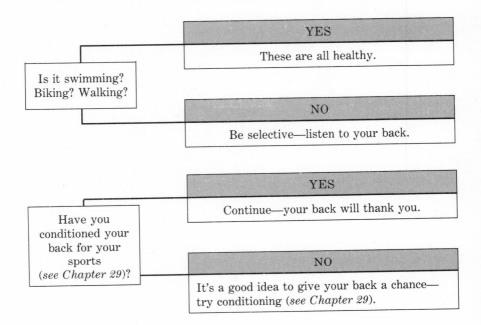

Is it swimming? Biking? Walking?

YES
These are all healthy.

NO
Be selective—listen to your back.

Have you conditioned your back for your sports (see Chapter 29)?

YES
Continue—your back will thank you.

NO
It's a good idea to give your back a chance—try conditioning (see Chapter 29).

MEDICAL BACK-UP—MILD PAIN 2

If the diagnosis is correct, you shouldn't need much medical supervision now, but you may need some—even though Back First Aid and Back Second Aid should keep most problems well in the background. There are a few backup items worth mentioning.

■ *Medication.* In rare cases, you may need something stronger than an occasional aspirin or Tylenol. Check with your doctor to see if he or she would recommend a stronger analgesic for special situations—e.g., to have on hand (just in case) when traveling, especially over *back* roads!

■ *Modalities.*
Hot packs (or hot tub or Jacuzzi)—whatever feels good is okay.
Massage—Stroking massage: Why not? If you can get somebody to do it for you. Deep pressure on a persistent trigger point can be helpful.

Traction—If you're an inverted traction user and find it helpful, and if you have checked on the eye, blood pressure, and heart problems with your doctor, then go ahead. If you use inverted traction occasionally and are not sure if it helps—it probably does not, so don't bother. If you follow the programs in this book, you will probably not find traction worth the additional cost or the bother.

■ *Manipulation*—You have probably learned from experience your own favorite twists (self-manipulation) such as the double Knee to Chest, the Knee Back, and the Advanced Pelvic Rotation exercises in Chapter 26, and with mild symptoms you would rarely gain by any additional maneuvers. If, however, it's *back* again and you are having a moderate flare-up, and if professional manipulation has previously been helpful, you may benefit from another treatment.

■ *Injections*—Only if you are in a flare-up (it's back again), and if the Back First Aid has not helped.

■ *Health Care Assistance*—Routine follow-up visits to your physician or therapist are a good idea to make sure that you are staying on track, performing your exercises properly, and using good back ergometric protection. If your back is against the wall psychologically, socially, sexually, or for whatever reason, it is a good idea to talk to your doctor or another health professional he/she has recommended and get appropriate counseling. "Use your head, not your back."

MEDICAL BACK-UP OPTIONS

Use these Medical Back-Up Options to help you prepare questions for your visit to your physician and other health professionals— if indeed you make that decision because of mild pain. (For *additional information on these topics, see Chapter 12.*)

TABLE 4   MEDICAL BACK-UP OPTIONS—⬦

	COMMENTS		
	USUALLY HELPFUL	SOMETIMES HELPFUL	POTENTIALLY DANGEROUS
Rest		X	
Medications		X*	
Corset or brace		X*	
Modalities for pain			
Heat	X		
Cold	X		
Massage		X*	
Traction		X*	
TNS (transcutaneous nerve stimulation)		X*	
Exercise	X		
Manipulation			X
Injections			
Narcotic			X*
Trigger points	X*		
Facet Joints		X*	
Epidural			X*
Health Care Assistance		X*	
Psychological/Social/Medical Counseling		X*	

*not usually necessary

MEDICAL BACK-UP DECISION CHECK LIST— ⬦

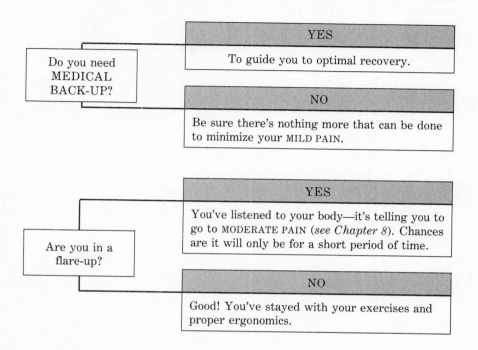

Do you need
MEDICAL
BACK-UP?

YES

To guide you to optimal recovery.

NO

Be sure there's nothing more that can be done to minimize your MILD PAIN.

Are you in a flare-up?

YES

You've listened to your body—it's telling you to go to MODERATE PAIN (*see Chapter 8*). Chances are it will only be for a short period of time.

NO

Good! You've stayed with your exercises and proper ergonomics.

CONCLUSION

In many ways, the milder the pain, the more difficult it is to deal with. The pain is there to tell us that something's not right and that we should take appropriate steps to minimize it. It's important to recognize that the pain is giving us a message and that to ignore the message may be to incur further back pain problems. By the same token, one can become morbidly concerned about every twinge and overreact, or even panic, as a consequence. We have to learn to distinguish between pain as a troublesome "hurt" and pain that is indicative of bodily harm. Obviously, not every twinge requires treatment, and equally obviously, as we are progressing with our exercises, we may incur some hurt and therefore need counsel as to whether we are risking harm. Nonetheless, when your pain is MILD, you have much more latitude in your activities and an even greater obligation to proceed with your exercise and conditioning so that the scope and satisfaction of life can be maximized and hopefully the pain level reduced to a minimum. When this happens, you're ready for Chapter 10, "Major Decisions for Minimal Pain, Level 1 Back Problems."

10.

MAJOR DECISIONS

FOR MINIMAL PAIN,

BACK PROBLEMS

Your back pain has healed for all intents and purposes—or perhaps it has never been any worse than it is now. Nonetheless, you may get an occasional reminder that the warranty on your back repair-job has some fine print. In this chapter we will provide you with information to make sure that warranty stays in force. In fact, the suggestions in this chapter on how to prevent back pain will apply to everyone, whether they have mild back pain now, have had it in the past, or have never had it and want to avoid getting it in the future. As you will see, most of what you need to think about if you're at MINIMAL PAIN, LEVEL 1 is just good common sense. But since good common sense isn't so common after all, the fine print in this section will help assure you that your back pain warranty is worth the paper that this is written on.

DECISION TREE— ○

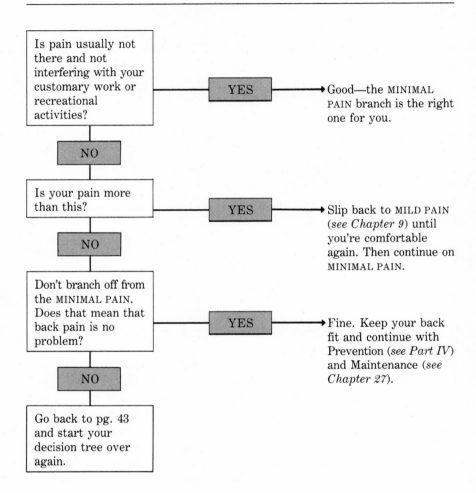

Is pain usually not there and not interfering with your customary work or recreational activities?

YES

Good—the MINIMAL PAIN branch is the right one for you.

NO

Is your pain more than this?

YES

Slip back to MILD PAIN (*see Chapter 9*) until you're comfortable again. Then continue on MINIMAL PAIN.

NO

Don't branch off from the MINIMAL PAIN. Does that mean that back pain is no problem?

YES

Fine. Keep your back fit and continue with Prevention (*see Part IV*) and Maintenance (*see Chapter 27*).

NO

Go back to pg. 43 and start your decision tree over again.

BACK HOME TREATMENT—MINIMAL PAIN 1

BACK FIRST AID

You don't need it now, but it may be good to know about it just in case. Use Chapter 6 (*see pg. 42*) as your guide if the need should arise.

BACK SECOND AID

■ *Rest.* See Back Second Aid Decision Check List, below.

■ *Back Protection Ergonomics.* Do your thing, but use your head and spare your back (*see Chapter 17*).

■ *Medications.* For what?

■ *Home Therapies.* O.K., if you want to indulge yourself (*see Chapter 15*).

■ *Assistance.* Don't ask for trouble—do ask for help if you need it (*see "Back Second Aid, General Assistance," pg. 63, in Chapter 8).*

■ *Diet.* Eat whatever you feel like as long as it is nutritious, non-constipating, and keeps you slim. If it's fattening—back away!

■ *Exercise.* See Back Second Aid Decision Check List, below.

BACK SECOND AID DECISION CHECK LIST—○

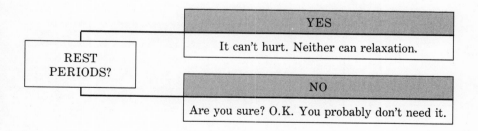

REST PERIODS?	YES
	It can't hurt. Neither can relaxation.
	NO
	Are you sure? O.K. You probably don't need it.

BACK SECOND AID DECISION CHECK LIST— ◯

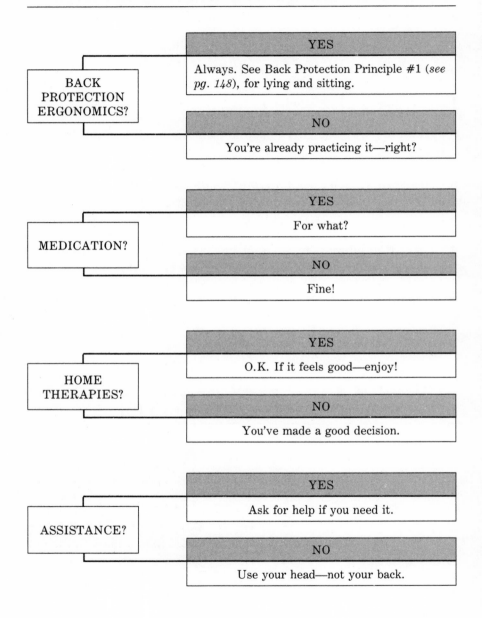

BACK PROTECTION ERGONOMICS?

YES

Always. See Back Protection Principle #1 (*see pg. 148*), for lying and sitting.

NO

You're already practicing it—right?

MEDICATION?

YES

For what?

NO

Fine!

HOME THERAPIES?

YES

O.K. If it feels good—enjoy!

NO

You've made a good decision.

ASSISTANCE?

YES

Ask for help if you need it.

NO

Use your head—not your back.

BACK SECOND AID DECISION CHECK LIST— ○

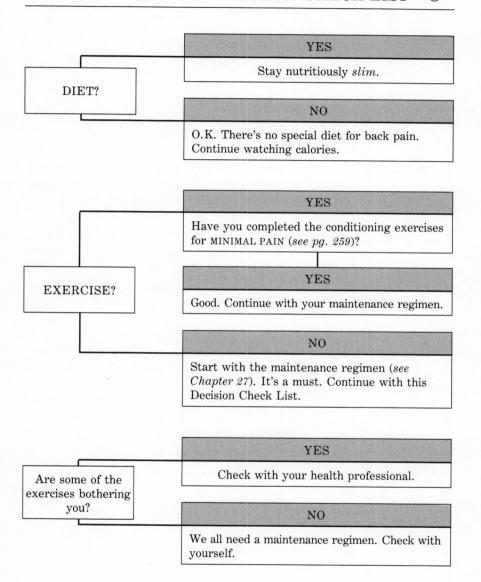

DIET?

YES

Stay nutritiously *slim*.

NO

O.K. There's no special diet for back pain. Continue watching calories.

EXERCISE?

YES

Have you completed the conditioning exercises for MINIMAL PAIN (*see pg. 259*)?

YES

Good. Continue with your maintenance regimen.

NO

Start with the maintenance regimen (*see Chapter 27*). It's a must. Continue with this Decision Check List.

Are some of the exercises bothering you?

YES

Check with your health professional.

NO

We all need a maintenance regimen. Check with yourself.

BACK-PROTECTED VIGOROUS EXERCISE— MINIMAL PAIN 1 *(see also Part V)*

■ *Cycling*—"Bike Back" hints *(see Chapter 29)* will keep you rolling along.

■ *Nautilus*—Use "Weights and Backs" guidelines *(see Chapter 29).*

■ *Swimming*—Anything goes, but be careful with the butterfly and with diving. Try to minimize arching your neck or back.

■ *Skiing*—Okay in the snow, but water skiing is a no-no. If you are not sure you're okay, take lessons. Check your bindings. Stay on good snow. No rope tows. Let's face it—you're still at risk.

■ *Walking and Jogging*—Walk vigorously and jog if you must, but wear well fitted, well made jogging shoes and try to run on soft, level turf. Avoid downhill jogging—walk if necessary. Running on a treadmill may be less jolting to your back. Remember that the twisting in race walking can be harder on your back than jogging.

■ *Tennis*—Take lessons and smooth out your strokes. Your serve may need to be modified to avoid excessive back bending. *(See "Stroke Back" in Chapter 29, pg. 280.)*

■ *Yoga*—can give you a good workout. Remember, it takes time and conditioning before you're ready for the more vigorous and demanding yoga exercises. Even if you've been with it for a long time, don't rush it. And if the exercise doesn't feel right for you—question it.

BACK-PROTECTED VIGOROUS SPORTS DECISION CHECK LIST— ◯

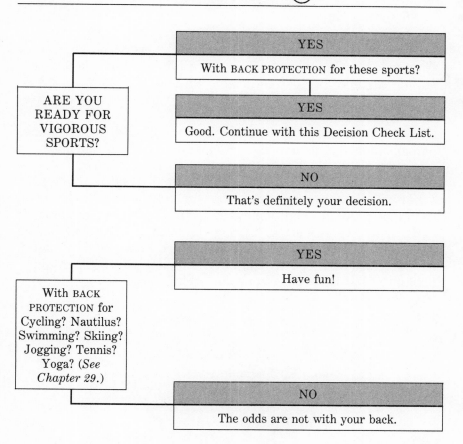

ARE YOU READY FOR VIGOROUS SPORTS?

> YES
> With BACK PROTECTION for these sports?

> YES
> Good. Continue with this Decision Check List.

> NO
> That's definitely your decision.

With BACK PROTECTION for Cycling? Nautilus? Swimming? Skiing? Jogging? Tennis? Yoga? (See Chapter 29.)

> YES
> Have fun!

> NO
> The odds are not with your back.

MEDICAL BACK-UP—MINIMAL PAIN ◯

■ *Medications.* If you are still on medication for your back, check with your doctor—he or she may have forgotten to tell you to quit.

■ *Corset or Brace.* Only if you need a security belt.

■ *Modalities for pain.* Professional therapy at this point is over-doing it. Whoever is paying the bills is being taken for a ride, unless you have had a set-*back*.

Traction—If you still like to hang upside down, why not! The "why not" means you've checked your eyes, heart, and blood pressure recently. If you haven't started traction, don't bother.

Massage—Enjoy!

■ *Exercise.* Your maintenance regimen, exercise, is your Back "Vitamin" (*see Chapter 27*). The "Five-Minute Back Saver" (*see Chapter 28*) may be just the right "vitamin" for you. (*See also Chapter 25, "Back Reconditioning."*) If you're feeling insecure, consult your health professional.

Special conditioning—Remember all of your other joints. Compensation for an improperly functioning knee, shoulder, or elbow may have to take place in the back, and then strain will be the name of your game. Get back into an old sport gradually. No pitcher will pitch nine innings in the summer without having gone through a gradual conditioning program in the spring. So, no matter what the season is, "spring" training is necessary before you get into competition. Warm-up before and cool-down after each exercise. Be S-A-F-E and have sufficient Strength, Agility, Flexibility, and Endurance for your athletic activity.

> S   Be STRONG enough
> A   AGILE enough
> F   FLEXIBLE enough
> E   have enough ENDURANCE
>   for exercise activities

■ *Manipulation.* If someone is still manipulating you, believe me, you're being manipulated. Stop this nonsense.

■ *Injections.* There's no excuse at this point. If it's *back* again, that's another story.

■ *Health Care Assistance.* If in doubt, get a check-up—an ounce of prevention is always a good buy.

MEDICAL BACK-UP OPTIONS

Use these Medical Back-Up Options to help you prepare questions for your visit to your physician and other health professionals—if indeed you make the decision that you have this need because of minimal pain. (*Additional information on these topics is in Chapter 12.*)

TABLE 5   MEDICAL BACK-UP OPTIONS— ○

	USUALLY HELPFUL	COMMENTS SOMETIMES HELPFUL	POTENTIALLY DANGEROUS
Rest		X*	
Medications		X*	
Corset or brace		X*	
Modalities for pain			
Heat	X*		
Cold	X*		
Massage		X*	
Traction		X*	
TNS (transcutaneous nerve stimulation)		X*	
Exercise	X		
Manipulation			X*
Injections			
Narcotic			X*
Trigger points	X*		
Facet Joints		X*	
Epidural			X*
Health Care Assistance		X*	
Psychological/Social/Medical Counseling		X*	

*not usually necessary

MEDICAL BACK-UP DECISION CHECK LIST— ○

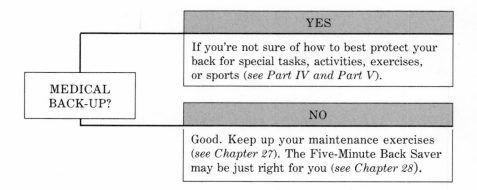

	YES
	If you're not sure of how to best protect your back for special tasks, activities, exercises, or sports (*see Part IV and Part V*).
MEDICAL BACK-UP?	
	NO
	Good. Keep up your maintenance exercises (*see Chapter 27*). The Five-Minute Back Saver may be just right for you (*see Chapter 28*).

CONCLUSION

MINIMAL PAIN, LEVEL 1 is a mixed blessing. If you started out with Severe Pain, Level 4 and you're now at Minimal Pain, Level 1, then it's clearly a blessing to have back discomfort at such a low level and relatively infrequently. If you've never had back pain, then even Minimal Level back pain is a nuisance at best and an all too clear reminder that something unsavory may be going on behind your back. It's clear that even at a mild pain level, or at a level of no pain, once you have a back problem, you'll stay ahead of the game if you maintain your back in good condition and avoid activities that are apt to exploit your back pain vulnerability. By the same token, it is fruitless to engage in chronic medication and a variety of well intended but unnecessary treatments, unless you want to do it for the sheer luxury of it all.

If you have now established the severity of your back pain problem and taken the appropriate Back First Aid and Back Second Aid steps, Medical Back-Up is now in order. Whatever the cause of your low back pain, and however severe it might be, a proper medical diagnosis is essential so that appropriate therapy can be initiated promptly and an optimal outcome assured. Let's read on in Part III and learn what kinds of medical care we should look for, who should provide it, and what we can expect from it.

III.

THE HEALTH CARE

TEAM, DIAGNOSIS,

AND TREATMENT

11.

THE BACK QUACK

IS

A SIDETRACK

During the course of evolution, one of the most feared yet most valuable sensations has been that of pain. Pain tells us that something is wrong. Our response to pain initiates a series of behavioral changes that protect us (as well as most of the animal kingdom) by modifying our course of action and maximizing the chance of our recovery from whatever injury or illness has provoked the pain. In the case of back pain, the intrusion of pain provides us literally with a "painful awareness" that we must do things differently in order to function and that we must take necessary action to get rid of the pain and restore our optimal level of function. That awareness should lead us to consider what kind of medical care is necessary, what kinds of health care professionals should be consulted, and what kinds of diagnostic procedures and treatments they can provide.

Because you are experiencing pain and impairment of function, you may be tempted to find a quick and unconventional solution to your problem. This chapter will give you some tips on how to avoid being taken in by false promises and phony cures.

"It's worth a try." Is it? "What can I lose?" Plenty!

When the realization dawns that back pain, like an unwanted out-of-town relative, has moved into your life and gives no obvious signs of leaving, you may get desperate. If you've been told that you need to rest, wear a corset, take pills, avoid strenuous activities, and do special exercises daily, you will be tempted to find a faster answer and an easier out. Admitting that you've really got to deal with your back problem may be so difficult that you try to deny its existence. This denial of serious problems or illnesses is a common phenomenon and can lead to tragic consequences. You do have something to lose, and there are a lot of quacks out there to help see to it that you lose it. Pain, fear, ignorance, and false hope set you up as a "mark" for larcenous charlatans to "sting." A billion-plus dollars a year line quacks' pockets and waste precious health care dollars.

Many back problems and other disorders ultimately heal themselves, but if you had just swallowed a "mega-mineral" and felt relieved of your pain—while your physician had not yet cured you—you would swear by it and tell all your friends about it. If you choked on alfalfa tablets and your back got worse, you wouldn't tell anyone. The power of belief in the magic of science (or of shamans) and faith in any treatment are powerful influences on our ability to withstand pain and suffering and can affect the actual course of many illnesses. Quacks know this all too well. They are prepared to take full advantage of your misplaced hope and your faith in their phony cures.

Someone always has, and always has had, something better that came from somewhere else. The Roman quacks "stung" with Egyptian and Chaldean "cures," Hippocrates worried about quacks in Greece before the Romans came into the picture. In the last century, if the Indians used it, it had to be good. Today, that still applies to yucca and other herbal remedies. Not only do so-called "innocent herbs" often come from exotic places, but purveyors of these "natural medicines" have been known to lace some of them with cortisone and Butazolidin to enhance their effects, with wanton disregard for the side effects. How, then, can rest and exercise, or surgery, compete with whatever is so new and so special that you can only get it in Mexico, Hong Kong, Las Vegas, or somewhere else?

The cost, the technology, and the sometimes impersonal nature of modern medical care tempts the more vulnerable and more gullible among us to seek an alternative treatment—some simple formula that demands little (except money) and promises much. *New* technology is particularly tempting for exploitation by charlatans. Benjamin Franklin's discovery of electricity led to a variety of electrical therapies, most of which have fallen by the wayside, but some of which are finding a place in contemporary medicine. Magnetism, copper bracelets, and even moon rocks have had their vogue in the past as pain relievers, and human nature being what it is, will probably be re-packaged and promoted in the future. A case in point is the laser technology that is being employed with great precision in a variety of procedures, but is offered without proof as a treatment in what is called laser acupuncture. Who knows—maybe laser acupuncture will work. The point is that no one knows, and until exotic therapeutic inventions are scientifically studied, they should be left alone by you.

How do you spot a quack or a quack book? You might find both in "health" food stores and the latter in your public library as well. The average public librarian is not well enough informed to distinguish between quackery and authentic medical information, and further, is prevented from making such distinctions, because of the quack's protection under the first amendment of our constitution.

Look out for simple answers to complex problems. The quack will seduce you with tranquilizing words to describe his or her therapy, words such as "safe," "quick," "easy," and "cure." He will quote "research" that has never been published in a credible medical journal, or that's out of date and long since refuted, to support his unique "breakthrough." To claim that a treatment for arthritis and back pain can utilize one simple approach (be it diet, exercise, herbs, or drugs) would presume that gout, lumbago, rheumatoid arthritis, osteoporosis, osteoarthritis, etc., are similar disorders all susceptible to the same simple cure. You might as well throw in baldness, hernias, kidney stones, impotence, and flat feet. But most of us are too sophisticated nowadays to fall for that.

The bottom line is that scientific breakthroughs are unlikely to come out of Madison Avenue. Don't let yourself be taken in: Back off and get proper medical care for your back.

12.

WHAT KIND OF

DOCTOR

SHOULD I SEE?

There is a saying that a doctor who diagnoses and treats himself has a fool for a patient and a fool for a doctor. The following material contains a series of problems that you and your medical doctor might consider in getting at what is causing, and therefore what might be done to help cure, your back pain. Unless your problem is short-lived or mild back pain, don't go it alone. Don't fool around.

FAMILY PHYSICIAN

Your *family physician* should be the first doctor you contact in any illness or injury, and this includes back pain. He can guide you to the necessary steps for proper relief and, when warranted, can help you select the proper consultant or therapist for specialized treatment. But what if you don't have a family physician and you do have severe back pain? The Back First Aid section in this book (*see pg. 44*) can help you to control the pain, and your local County Medical Association can help you find a family physician to assist you. There are also many small clinics that offer emergency care, but not all of them provide consistent high-quality care. If you have no alternative but to seek emergency room treatment, you will probably have a better chance receiving high-quality care if you go to the emergency room of a major hospital known to have a highly respected medical and surgical staff.

MEDICAL SPECIALISTS

SURGICAL SPECIALISTS

What kinds of *medical specialists* treat back pain? When you have back pain, it is possible to have several different kinds of doctors who might "work behind your back." In addition to the pain, suffering, and worry about how to stay on the job, which back pain can provoke, there lurks behind every back pain the possibility that a surgical procedure, with its attendant risks, may be required. Therefore, the first physician to see in the event of a back pain, all things being equal, is probably not a physician who does back surgery. Why not? It has been said that to the man who has a hammer in his hand, everything starts to look like a nail. It has been said that to a physician trained in surgery, the solution to an illness or injury tends to be biased toward surgical procedures (substitute scalpel for hammer) rather than more conservative medical approaches. So, although both *orthopedic surgeons* (orthopods) and *neurosurgeons* may have great skill in performing back surgery when needed, by and large they do not have as great an interest in attending to the less glamorous details of a conservative treatment that might assure a successful nonsurgical outcome.

There are, of course, many exceptions to the above general statement, and in particular there are outstanding orthopedic surgeons who have made great contributions to our understanding of the value of conservative care for back pain. Further, it goes without saying that if you have to have back surgery, it should be done by a surgeon who regularly does spinal surgery, to assure that he or she has both good surgical judgment and outstanding surgical technical skills.

The *orthopedic surgeon* is a surgeon who is trained to deal with bones, muscles, and joints; with fractures, sprains, and bone tumors; and with the correction of skeletal deformities. Pain in skeletal structures, particularly that requiring surgical treatment, is what brings the orthopedist to the back pain problem. Many orthopedists develop great skill in dealing with back pain problems, as well as in the surgical treatment of back pain. The skill and dexterity of a surgeon in handling the delicate nervous tissues of the spinal cord and the nerves that branch from it are dependent on the interests and specialized abilities of the surgeon. This point is critical in that, in times past, most disk surgery was performed by *neurosurgeons*, whose training is particularly focused on the handling of delicate nerve structures. Many neurosurgeons are highly skilled in the management of back surgery, but often the mechanical aspects of back pain that are of concern to the orthopedic surgeon are not particularly emphasized in the training of the neurosurgeon. In the final analysis, highly trained and experienced orthopedic surgeons and neurosurgeons can be equally skilled in the surgical treatment of lumbar disk problems. Certainly, where the orthopedic mechanical aspects of the problem predominate, the orthopedic surgeon is the better choice. When there are delicate nerve tissues, perhaps tissues injured in a previous surgery, or where there is a question of a possible tumor or other disorder affecting the nerve, then the neurosurgeon becomes the consultant of choice. In many instances, both neurosurgeons and orthopedists work together on complicated back surgery problems.

It's your back. Look over your shoulder and be sure that the surgeon who is working back there is not gaining surgical experience at your expense.

REHABILITATION SPECIALISTS

The nonsurgical specialty that is most attuned to conservative treatment of back pain is probably one of the least known of the medical specialties: *Physical Medicine and Rehabilitation* or *PM&R*. The physicians who are specialists in physical medicine and rehabilitation are called *physiatrists* (*phys* for physical as opposed to *psych* for psychological, as in psychiatrist) and are knowledgeable in exercise therapy and in the use of posture, back protection, pain avoidance measures, as well as *physical* agents such as electricity, heat, cold, etc., for treatment. As with all specialists, there are those with greater skills in some areas than in others, so physiatrists who primarily treat stroke cases may not be particularly competent in the management of spinal disorders.

■ *Rheumatologists*. Rheumatologists are specialists in Internal Medicine and in the treatment of arthritic disorders. They are particularly skilled in diagnosing medical conditions and arthritic disorders that may affect the spine. Those rheumatologists who have been trained in the tradition of British rheumatology, where rehabilitation and medical orthopedic treatment are strongly emphasized, are usually very skillful in the conservative management of back pain. This is true of many rheumatologists trained in the United States. Unfortunately, however, the bulk of their training has emphasized the problems dealing with inflamed joints, and the general body systemic illnesses that also affect joints, rather than the common disk-related low back pain disorders.

■ *Osteopaths*. Osteopaths today are trained in conventional medical practices as well as in the use of manipulation (*see Chapter 14*) in the treatment of muscle and skeletal disorders. Many osteopaths are family physicians and use manipulation to treat neck, back, and other joint disorders selectively for their own patients. Others primarily treat neck and back problems, and still others specialize in the various medical and surgical specialties of modern medicine. The osteopathic physician with a special interest in conservative treatment of back pain can provide useful assistance to a back pain sufferer.

■ *Chiropractors*. Chiropractors are the other group of practitioners who advocate manipulation and "hands on" (manual) therapies for back pain. Chiropractic training and licensing does not permit the prescription of medicine or the use of injections or surgery by chiropractors. Since the role of manipulation in the treatment of back pain is a limited one, and since the medical (and lack of surgical) education of chiropractors does not include the full scope of modern medical school training, a referral to a chiropractor probably is best utilized only in cases of low back pain of short duration and moderate severity where there is a possibility that manipulation may help speed the recovery.

■ *Physical Therapist* (P.T.). A P.T. is trained in the use of a variety of physical (nonmedical) treatments including heat, cold, electricity, ultrasound, traction, massage, and exercise. Some physical therapists are trained in the use of various combinations of massage and manipulation called mobilization, muscle energy techniques, or manual therapies. The physical therapist can be extremely helpful in the treatment of back disorders if she/he has had appropriate training and experience in the treatment of these conditions and works closely with and under the prescription of a physician knowledgeable in the management of back conditions.

■ *Occupational Therapist* (O.T.) The O.T. who has been trained in assisting patients with back pain can be invaluable in teaching the proper techniques for lying, sitting, standing, lifting, bending, driving, traveling, and even making love. All of these activities of daily living (ADL) need to be performed in such a manner as to allow us to do what we must do without aggravating our back pain problems. Usually affiliated with major hospitals and/or rehabilitation clinics, occupational therapists are not available in all communities. And, as in all specialties, there are many occupational therapists who have had no particular training or experience in the management of back pain disorders. *Caveat emptor*—let the buyer beware.

HOLISTIC MEDICINE

What about a *holistic* approach? The term holistic comes from the word "whole," which implies a concern for the totality of the patient's medical, psychological, physical, social, economic, and environmental needs. Clearly, all of these factors play a role in any illness and are important to some extent in every case of low back pain. The implication of a holistic approach is that all the various factors that play a direct or indirect role in the suffering of the back pain patient warrant consideration and, where needed, intervention by health care professionals with the appropriate expertise. When this involves various combinations of the health professions previously described, with each professional performing his or her role as coordinated and directed by the physician in charge, one can have the best of a holistic approach.

The holistic approach can, in some instances, be expanded to include specialists trained in psychological and social or vocational counseling, in yoga, in dietary instruction for weight control, and possibly in acupuncture for pain control. The most important thing about holistic medicine is to see to it that there is a physician in the center of the hole. The physician should guide, coordinate, and advise the various contributors to this holistic endeavor so that the proper integration of less traditional medical approaches with conventional medical practice can provide the whole patient with the optimum benefit. The alternative is an unholy, mindless spinning of misguided wheels, which can lead the patient and his or her back down a painfully wrong path to greater suffering.

13.

JUST TESTING

We live in a highly technical age, and there is no doubt that modern technology has opened vast frontiers in medical science. But we can be overwhelmed by technology and over-sold on tests. The "good" tests, which we will discuss in this chapter— CAT scan, EMG, MRI (magnetic resonance imaging), or myelogram —are about 80 to 90% accurate in good hands. So the tests give information that can be erroneous, and even when correct, must be properly interpreted. Since everyone over 50 years of age has disk disease to some extent, a CAT scan, MRI, or myelogram will predictably show abnormalities in persons over 50. But what do these abnormalities mean in *your* case? Will a decision that affects *your* low back pain be made? Yes, at times; and no, at other times. In fact, most back pain and disk sufferers don't need such tests, because they respond to conservative treatment, and these tests really offer little if anything to the conduct of that treatment.

THE BETTER THE DOCTOR, THE FEWER THE TESTS

A skilled physician is like a good oil geologist. The latter knows the lay of the land and where to start digging for oil. The astute physician understands your back problem and knows when it is useful to order tests and what tests to order—and if he does not, he knows to request a consultation.

If you are in good health and/or recently had a checkup, you may already have most of the information you need, so be prepared to obtain a record of any relevant recent medical consultation, lab test, hospital visit, or X-ray before you see your doctor. If you have recent X-rays of your back and they were of good quality, then no further tests may be needed; a diagnosis can be established and a treatment plan initiated. In fact, one of the great challenges of medicine is that a treatment plan must be initiated by the doctor before all of the information required to make a diagnosis can be gathered. An illness is an evolving process. It may suggest certain conditions at one phase, only to declare its true nature later on. Sometimes we may have an illness that will run its course and leave without ever revealing its true nature. Was it a virus? A strain? A cramp? Your doctor will likely gather sufficient information, chart a course, and then assess your response to treatment before determining the need for more tests.

X-RAY

What is sufficient information? Again, if you are in apparent good health, but have developed low back pain, and you have none of the Danger Signals (*see pg. 26*), yet you fail to improve after two or three weeks, an X-ray of your lumbar spine is in order. The X-ray will reveal any evidence of arthritis, spinal developmental defects such as spondylolisthesis, or disk deterioration.

You should know that the soft tissues of the actual disk or the bulging of a protruding disk cannot be seen on conventional X-rays, and, in fact, can only be poorly visualized with the most modern MRI or CAT scans available. What can be seen on ordinary X-rays is a narrowing of the space between two vertebrae due to shrinking of the disk. The fact is that *routine X-rays* usually indicate only what has gone in the past—i.e., that the disk has been wearing out—but not what is going on now, unless a recent fracture (this should not be a surprise) or a bone disease or arthritis or a tumor is detected.

So why bother? A good question! Sometimes, albeit rarely,

useful information is gleaned from X-rays, and often medical-legal considerations influence the need for X-rays. But most often, the obvious is confirmed—that if you have gray hair or wrinkles, your spine will show some evidence of wear-and-tear in the disks and in the facet joints, and if you are a postmenopausal woman, the older you are, the more likely you are to see evidence of osteoporosis. Nonetheless, at this state of the art, spinal X-rays are the initial diagnostic test.

BLOOD AND URINE TESTS

If there is any question about your health status, or if you have been taking pain-killers or other medications, the status of your health and your susceptibility to more serious drug reactions will require a CBC (*complete blood count*) in which both your red and white blood cells are looked at and counted. The amount of hemoglobin or iron-containing pigment in your red cells is also determined, and the appearance of your blood platelets (*clotting particles*) is noted. Oftentimes a *sedimentation rate* is measured. This tests for inflammation in your system, which can be due to a variety of causes, such as inflammatory arthritis, infection, or malignancy, but it does not tell which is the cause. It is a simple test in which a column of blood is placed in a tube and the red and white cells are allowed to settle to the bottom for one hour. The rate at which these cells settle depends on how clumped they are. When there is some inflammation in your system, various factors in the blood cause the cells to clump more and therefore to settle more rapidly—this is an elevated sedimentation rate.

A *urine* sample is tested to rule out kidney or bladder problems that may be a factor in back pain. A gynecological examination and a Pap smear may also be required, depending on the symptoms. Clearly, before any tests are done, a careful history of your case and a complete examination should be done to uncover any otherwise unsuspected problems that could be contributing to your low back pain.

Another test—actually a panel of tests—that is often obtained at this stage of investigation is a blood *chemistry panel*. This blood test usually includes tests for calcium, phosphorus, sugar, protein, uric acid, bilirubin, sodium, potassium, chloride, creatinine (a measure of kidney function), and certain enzymes (chemical reaction expeditors) that reflect the workings of your liver, muscles, and bone. One enzyme, serum acid phosphatase, when elevated, is an indication of the spread of cancer from the prostate gland. Tests for thyroid function may be included because low thyroid function can be associated with generalized aching; excessive thyroid activity may cause osteoporosis; and both high and low thyroid activity can contribute to bone and muscle aching and muscle weakness.

At this point your doctor is reasonably sure that your general health is good and that you are likely to have a so-called discogenic basis (related to disk strain, or facet joint strain) for your low back pain. If your symptoms suggest otherwise, or if these tests indicate that you are not as healthy as you appear or that medications you have taken for your back pain or any other condition are disturbing your bodily functions, further medical diagnosis may be necessary. Sometimes a laboratory makes mistakes and tests that are abnormal, when repeated, turn out to be normal. So the first step oftentimes is to repeat any abnormal tests. Sometimes stopping the use of a medication will restore the blood tests to normal. Clearly, this requires careful judgment by your physician, because no medicine crucial to your well-being should be discontinued without careful consideration of the consequences. Obviously, you must tell your doctor what medications, vitamins, and even "health supplements" you are taking, for whatever reason, if he/she is to give the proper interpretation of your problem.

HOW ABOUT TESTS FOR ARTHRITIS?

Most often when you are told that you have severe arthritis in your spine, you don't! The likelihood is that your disks are wearing down and losing their shock-absorbing function, and as a natural consequence, you are adding bone around the edges of your vertebrae. These bony ridges may be quite prominent on X-rays of your spine, and they tend to look like spurs of bone. It is not hard to imagine one of these "spurs" jabbing into you like a thorn, but it is well to remember that a wise Mayo Clinic orthopedic surgeon once said, "You can't read the ouches on the X-rays." Actually, these so-called spurs or bone growths, called *osteophytes* (meaning "bone growth"), are blunt ridges, not sharp spurs, and rarely cause pain per se. Since it takes about six months for an osteophyte to form, it stands to reason, if you've had your symptoms for three months and you have huge osteophytes on your X-rays, that they were there long before you started hurting— and will still be there long after you have stopped hurting. You can't get rid of osteophytes by diet, vitamin therapy, or exercise, but weight loss if you are heavy, proper use of back protective body mechanics (as discussed in Part IV), localized pain control measures (e.g., cold packs, electrical stimulation, etc.), and proper reconditioning exercises (*see Chapter 26*) can get rid of the pain. So there is *good news for bad backs!*

When these wear-and-tear changes occur in the facet joints, one can get a true wear-and-tear osteoarthritis in these small joints. Even in relatively young adults, the facet joints may undergo wear-and-tear deterioration when the associated disks are no longer functioning properly. Osteoarthritis does not spread over your body—it stays where there has been excessive wear and tear. These osteoarthritic joints can ache and can cause stiffness from time to time, especially with unusual strain such as might occur from pulling weeds—a classic cause of the "crab grass back."

Occasionally, however, these osteophytes become large enough to squeeze one of the spinal nerves and cause nerve root irritation. When one osteoarthritic facet joint is the seat of unrelenting back discomfort, injections of cortisone-like drugs in relatively small amounts can often give relief. Rarely, a procedure is done in which the actual nerves that supply the affected facet joint (and usually the joint above and below) are interrupted either surgically, by cautery, or by the injection of chemicals that destroy these nerves. Unfortunately, these procedures do not have a particularly high success rate, and the cut or destroyed nerves tend to regenerate so that pain will eventually recur.

So much for wear and tear—what about real arthritis? The classic crippling arthritis that comes to mind is called *rheumatoid arthritis*. This typically affects joints all over the body, and in the neck in some cases, but not in the rest of the spine. So tests that attempt to determine the presence of something called *rheumatoid factor* and tests for other so-called connective tissue disorders, such as *systemic lupus erythematosus* (which affects joints and, often as not, the skin, eyes, throat, heart, lungs, and kidneys, but almost never the back) are usually a waste of time and money.

There is *one true arthritic disorder* that affects the spine: *ankylosing spondylitis* (a painful inflammatory joint disease that affects the spine and causes a bony bridging to occur between the vertebrae, thereby ankylosing or fusing portions of the spine). It can be suspected if the blood sedimentation rate is elevated (although it can actually be found in patients who have a normal sedimentation rate). There are several other diseases that are associated with arthritis in various joints and ankylosing spondylitis: Reiter's syndrome, colitic arthritis, psoriasis, and arthritis. None of these disorders has a blood test more specific than the sedimentation rate to identify it. Ankylosing spondylitis is diagnosed by finding characteristic arthritis changes in the sacroiliac joints. Sometimes these are difficult to see, and the newer CAT scan techniques may help. In any event, 90% of white patients with ankylosing spondylitis have a specific protein on the surface of their white blood cells (*leukocytes*) called B-27, which is detectable on a special blood test. This test is occasionally useful in diagnosing ankylosing spondylitis and the other disorders associated with a similar arthritic process in the spine. Remember that 10% of white people with ankylosing spondylitis do not have the B-27 protein on their white blood cells, and in other racial groups with ankylosing spondylitis the percentage is even higher. So there are lots of folks with ankylosing spondylitis who are B-27 negative (don't have it on the leukocytes) and lots more folks who are B-27 positive and are perfectly well. The point is that B-27 positivity only identifies a *susceptibility* to ankylosing spondylitis and certain related conditions, but it does not mean that you've got it or that you will get it in the future.

TESTING FOR TUMORS

Another blood test that is sometimes useful, when a rare bone cancer, *multiple myeloma*, is suspected as the cause of low back pain, is *serum protein electrophoresis*. This tells whether or not your body is manufacturing abnormal amounts of antibody-containing protein. This test and its refinements are used when multiple myeloma is suspected, but there are typically other clues on the X-rays, on urine tests, and also in the blood.

All of these tests may be inconclusive and lead to further

study by specialists. When there is uncertainty as to whether or not multiple myeloma or another form of cancer might be present, a *bone scan* may be ordered. In a bone scan, radioactive chemicals (*isotopes*) are injected into your veins. The chemical isotopes accumulate in bones or joints and can be counted by a Geiger-counterlike device. Abnormally high or low counts may indicate malignant growths in bone or, on occasion, a fracture undetected by X-ray. These bone scans also detect new bone growth occurring in osteophytes in otherwise normal patients with some disk degeneration. So these tests also require careful analysis and interpretation. A "positive" bone scan (one showing a so-called hot spot where isotopes are concentrated) may only be indicating new bone formation in an osteophyte developing around a worn disk. In addition to these diagnostic procedures, *computerized axial tomography* (CAT) scanning and *magnetic resonance imaging* (MRI) are powerful tools to help identify tumors in and around the spine. You will learn more about CAT scanning and MRI in the next section, on the war of nerves—testing for sciatica.

THE WAR OF NERVES—TESTING FOR SCIATICA

When low back pain is complicated by nerve root compression (*see "Serious Sciatica and Pinched Nerves," pg. 31*), there is a battle to be won. This is not "nervousness," but a pressure-irritation of the nerve root due to protrusion of a disk sufficient to pinch the nerve root. This nerve irritation usually causes enough discomfort to make you at the very least a bit nervous. It will also worry your doctor, who will test you with pins and brushes and check your reflexes to see if there is any loss of sensation, and if so, where. Your doctor will test the strength of your muscles to detect any weakness resulting from nerve root compression. He or she will also put you on your back, straighten out your good leg on the bed, and then lift your affected leg, keeping the knee straight. This is to see if the straight-leg sciatic-nerve stretch test causes leg pain (back pain does not count) during the first 30 degrees of elevation—which is an almost certain sign of sciatic nerve irritation. This test, called the Lasegue test (after Ernest Charles Lasegue, a French doctor who first described it), becomes less reliable as the straight leg is raised to 60 degrees or more, but it still gives a clear warning that more than just a back strain may be present. Patients with tight hamstrings (the muscles that stretch from their attachment in the buttocks to form cords or strings on either side of the back of the knee) may get a burning sensation in the back of the thigh at 60 degrees or so, but this does not necessarily mean nerve root compression. When the discomfort elicited by the Lasegue test spreads beyond the knee to the calf or foot, or when sciatic symptoms of tingling and pain are felt beyond the knee, there is a greater likelihood that sciatic nerve root compression exists.

A similar test, described by Dr. Leonard Wheeler Ely, stretches the nerve roots that join to form the femoral nerve, which supplies the muscles and tissues on the fronts of the thighs. These nerve roots are affected in only 2% of patients, so the Ely test is often omitted when there is obvious evidence of sciatic nerve root compression. The femoral nerve and one of its roots (usually the lowest, or 4th lumbar) are particularly suspect if your knee jerk reflex is weak, since the femoral nerve carries the message that makes the knee jerk reflex react.

The Ely or femoral nerve root stretch test is usually performed by having you lie face down and then bending your knee, so that your foot approaches your buttock. Your thigh is then raised to see if pain in the front of the thigh can be produced. The muscles in the fronts of the thighs (the quadriceps muscles) are, like the hamstring muscles, often somewhat tight and painful when stretched; so in both the Ely and the Lasegue tests, both legs are compared, to be sure that there is a true abnormality.

When nerve root compression is diagnosed, the treatment plan can be initiated without more elaborate confirmation unless something peculiar or dangerous is suspected. This is possible because over 80% of patients with sciatic or femoral nerve root pressure due to disk protrusions will recover without surgery—if properly treated. If, however, more than one nerve root is apparently involved, or if nerve roots on both sides of the body are affected, a large, potentially dangerous disk protrusion, or worse, a tumor, has to be suspected, and this will require further testing. Needless to say, if you are losing control of your bowel and/or bladder, or are having great difficulty in urinating, a large disk protrusion or tumor must be suspected, and it is likely that surgery will be required.

When symptoms suggest a potentially dangerous condition

such as a tumor or a massive disk protrusion, the two most reliable and least injurious tests are the CAT scan and the MRI scan. CAT stands for computerized axial tomography, and this highly sophisticated computer-assisted X-ray gives a three-dimensional view of the spine and other structures with no more X-ray exposure than that of a conventional X-ray. A CAT scan is an expensive test, but it does not ordinarily require any injections, and it will readily detect most tumors or disk protrusions. Where CAT scanners are not available, a *myelogram* may be necessary. This involves injecting an iodine-containing dye into the spinal canal. The dye (sometimes air is also used) creates a sharp black-and-white contrast with the bone and nerve tissue. What appear to be bumps along the spinal nerves or the dural sac (a hard connective-tissue sac that surrounds and protects the spinal cord and nerve roots) are an indication of something—disk or tumor—pressing against these nerve structures. With small tumors or disk protrusions, a myelogram will occasionally provide information not obtained by the CAT scan, and even more information when it is performed immediately prior to the CAT scan. However, this is becoming less and less the case, as CAT scanners and the latest diagnostic aid, the MRI scan, become more and more sophisticated.

The MRI (magnetic resonance imager), also called NMR (nuclear magnetic resonance scanner) is the latest and potentially most sophisticated computerized device for three dimensional visualization of body tissues. It even has the capability of recording some of the chemical reactions that are taking place in the body. It consists of a powerful magnet, which encircles the patient and causes the hydrogen atoms in the body's tissues to emit a detectable radio wave. The concentration of hydrogen atoms is greater or lesser, depending on how much water (H_2O) is present in the tissue. The force of the magnetic field can be varied. This and the concentration of hydrogen will create differences in the radio signal's intensity from each body organ or tissue, such as the spinal cord or the surrounding fat. The sophisticated computer can then analyze from the radio signal the pattern and shape of the tissue, such as the spinal cord, that is giving off that signal. The MRI can outline non-bony structures such as the disk, the spinal nerves, or the surrounding fat quite well, but it does not image bony structures.

It is important to remember that the MRI gives a picture

that is very useful and is the next best thing to seeing the actual structures, as during surgery. The MRI has the advantage that no X-ray exposure is involved. It has thus far been a safe procedure for examining a variety of body structures including the brain, eyes, heart, lungs, and digestive organs, as well as the spinal cord. The major danger is that magnetizable metallic fragments can be dislodged. Therefore, patients with bone plates, or implants such as the metal in a hip joint replacement, can be injured by the magnet. An MRI examination is also moderately more expensive at this time than a CAT scan, but as more MRIs become available, the cost will probably become more competitive.

In fact, one can see so much pathology on a CAT or MRI scan that its use may actually lead to over-diagnosis, over-treatment, and ultimately, excessive surgery. Physicians will have to learn how to correlate the "ouches" not only with conventional X-rays but the more sophisticated and more detailed information of a CAT or MRI scan.

The point is that by the time we are 50 years old, we all have at least minor disk and facet joint abnormalities. Now, most of us are not hurting, so it is obvious that a lot of detectable abnormality has nothing to do with symptoms. Almost everyone over 50 would see cause for alarm if they had a lumbar CAT or MRI scan, because some bulging of the lower spinal disks is likely to be noted, as is wear-and-tear narrowing of the adjacent facet joints with bony osteophyte formation. Similar wear-and-tear changes in sacroiliac joints are also regularly seen. The CAT and MRI scans are a little like a magnifying glass view of your chin. All of a sudden there are all kinds of bumps, warts, ingrown hairs, pimples, and blackheads that you never noticed before. The magnified skin looks like a disaster area, yet you know it to be "normal," even though you can see all of the abnormalities with magnification. Similarly, the CAT and MRI scans show a lot of bumps and scars, which are not truly normal, but from the standpoint of contributing to any detectable symptoms, are of no consequence.

In summary, large disk protrusions and, of course, tumors detected by CAT scan, myelogram, or MRI are likely to be important causes of important symptoms, and obviously they may require surgical treatment. Small tumors may also require surgical treatment, but small disk protrusions and swelling, even with nerve pressure or conditions that aggravate osteoarthritic facet joints, are all likely to heal without surgery—and should be given every chance to do so!

ANYTHING ELSE TO TEST FOR NERVE ROOT COMPRESSION?

Any doctor worth his or her salt can think of another test or two to do. But there are two tests that tell us something about how your nerves and muscles are working that can be helpful in sorting out disk and nerve root problems. These tests are called *nerve conduction velocity* (NCV) and *electromyography* (EMG).

NCV is performed by using an electrical stimulator. Electrodes, taped to the skin, send a message down a nerve to a recording electrode. The recording electrode is also taped to the skin or sometimes attached by a needle under the skin. The rate at which the message travels down the nerve and the intensity of the recorded electrical response determine how well the nerve is working and if there are blockages along its course. EMG is performed by inserting fine needles into muscles. The electrical discharge of muscles at rest and during contraction can be heard over an amplifier and seen and photographed on an electronic monitoring device called an *oscilloscope*. Abnormalities of muscle function due to damaged nerve supply or muscle disease can be readily detected with this technique. In obvious cases of sciatic and femoral nerve root impairment, simple tests that your doctor performs in his or her office (pinprick, brushing your skin, reflex hammer test, muscle strength test, straight leg raising) usually suffice for diagnosis, and treatment can be commenced directly.

Sometimes the findings at the bedside are confusing. There may be two disorders in the same patient (the patient may have diabetes affecting the nerves in his legs and a sciatic nerve root that is pinched by a disk). Sometimes a nerve on the inside of the ankle is pinched under a band of tissue at a place called the *tarsal* (ankle) *tunnel*; and rarely, other nerves, pinched at various places in the leg or damaged by illness or injury, cause difficulty in the interpretation of your signs and symptoms.

There are other diseases that affect nerves and muscles besides those mentioned, so the combination of nerve and muscle testing by NCV and EMG may be very important to help clarify a confusing diagnostic picture. However, these electrical tests are somewhat uncomfortable and relatively expensive. Where simple bedside clinical testing provides an adequate explanation of your symptoms, additional tests are not required for the proper planning of your treatment. Remember that most cases of nerve root compression due to disk pressure recover without surgery and without *chymopapain enzyme treatment* either (*see Chapter 16*).

SEP

The latest innovation in electrodiagnosis involves stimulating a nerve in the lower leg and recording the intensity of the response in the brain. This is done by means of small electrodes that are pasted on the scalp. This technique is called SEP— *somatosensory* (body nerves for transmitting feeling) *evoked potentials* (electrical activity recorded in the brain when a nerve is stimulated). It is new, safe, and expensive. Its potential value lies in the determination of the extent of nerve root or spinal cord malfunction due to a pinching effect on the spinal nerves in a narrow spinal canal in an otherwise equivocal case of spinal stenosis (*see pg. 31*).

THERMOGRAPHY

A relatively new test that has been introduced in the assessment of back pain is called *thermography*. Liquid crystals (made from cholesterol) used for thermography (LCT) are sensitive to small variations in temperature and turn a specific color at a specific temperature. These crystals are impregnated into plastic sheets and made into pillows that can be pressed against the body to detect changes in skin temperature. Normally, there are variations in skin temperature over different parts of the body, but they are symmetrical. In the presence of nerve root irritation, the skin supplied by the injured nerve root will be at a lower temperature than adjacent skin or skin on the opposite side. Skin overlying trigger areas in fibrositis (*see pg. 24*) may initially be warmer and later cooler than surrounding skin. Because these painful trigger points are so often overlooked on examination and can be detected, or at least suspected, from thermography, there has been an inference that thermograms provide a picture of pain—in color! This is a gross exaggeration and has caused thermography to become something of a diagnostic hot potato. Although still controversial, thermograms are now being used (and sometimes misused) in the courtroom in an attempt to provide jurors with what is purported to be a "visual image" of the claimant's pain.

Thermograms offer little to a skilled physician, but not all physicians are skilled in examining for trigger points or subtle changes in nerve root function, so thermography may find a place as a diagnostic tool. Some physicians may find it useful to use thermograms in order to take a second look at "neurotic" patients who keep complaining about their back pain or sciatic pain without apparent cause. They may be neurotic, but they may have cause!

14.

MANIPULATION:

WHAT'S "IN"

AND

WHAT'S "OUT"?

When there is an abrupt change from a relatively normal-feeling back ("I didn't even know I had a back . . .") to a very painful or stiff spine, which often forces us to walk bent over or tilted to one side, we say, "My back went out." Unfortunately, when the back "goes out," it does not go anywhere, and usually when this occurs, we're not going anywhere either—certainly not out on the town! Well, what's "out" if it's out, and how do we get it back in? This question is a source of serious debate and, not infrequently, of acrimonious argument.

WHAT'S "OUT" WHEN THE BACK GOES OUT?

No one argues over whether a sprained disk can swell and bulge and press on nerves. No one argues (because of the ample evidence at surgery) over whether part of the central portion of the disk, the nucleus pulposus, can bulge through a tear in the surrounding annulus fibrosus ligaments and at times cause pressure on the sciatic nerve (*see pg. 13; Fig. 8*). But there is a lot of argument about what happens next. No one can observe the

119

healing phase of a "sprained" disk because even the most sophisticated diagnostic devices (X-ray, ultrasound, MRI or CAT scans; *see Chapter 13*) cannot yet visualize this healing process. Most of us over 50 years of age have disks that have become shrunken in the center and partially protrude around the edges, between the vertebrae. These deformed but painless disks provide eloquent testimony to the healing response to previous normal daily wear and tear or disk injuries: Whether in previous times there was a phase of gross injury and visible swelling that has healed can only be guessed at.

Anyone who has smashed a thumb or stubbed a big toe knows what a swollen, throbbing thing that is. The big toe is "out" of the shoe and the thumb is kept "out" of the handshake. These are temporary, reversible injuries that typically heal with complete restoration of normal structure and function to the toe or thumb. Presumably, much of the injury and swelling that occurs with low back disk or facet joint sprains and strains heals as well. The swollen "out" part heals and shrinks into a near-normal state, with perhaps a minor, and sometimes major, but no longer painful bulge of scar tissue as the only residual trace of the disk injury.

It is obvious that you cannot push the bulging swelling of a smashed thumb or toe back into anything. Protecting these injured structures from further injury allows nature to do the healing and relieve the swelling. Patience and protection, nature and nurture, get the job done. But we all know of someone whose back has "gone out" and then, either as a result of a sudden twist, or more impressively, by a manipulation procedure, the back has "gone back in." This phenomenon, which has served as a basis for manipulation treatment by lay manipulators, bone setters, osteopaths, and chiropractors, cannot be denied. What is going on back there?

MANIPULATION—WHEN PUSH COMES TO SHOVE

THE "INS" AND THE "OUTS"

Disk problems are quite rare in childhood. Children are generally very supple and their disks are efficient shock absorbers. Young disks contain relatively more of the viscous material in the nucleus pulposus and absorb more water into the center of the disk. The relatively large, turgid yet pliable disks of young adults can be contrasted with the shrunken, more rigid disks of the middle and advanced years. The former resemble dried cereal soaked in cream; the latter clearly could use more cream. In fact, these "dry" shrunken disks account for most of the loss of height we experience as we grow older.

Because the disks of young adults have a very gooey nucleus pulposus center, their disk injuries characterized by annulus fibrosus ligament tears behave differently from the injuries in older disks. The gooey material in younger disks tends to push through the torn ring fibers and bulge into weak spots on either side of the back fibrous rings of the annular ligament. This creates a kind of thick wedge between two vertebrae that can cause one vertebra to tilt forward and often to one or the other side of the one below. When this has happened and we stand upright, we look like we are bending forward or tilting to one side or both. We tend to bend as a consequence of the wedging effect and also because we lean to the side away from areas of pressure on injured ligaments, joints, or nerves. Whichever way we're bending, we are bent out of shape and the back is "out."

WHAT'S "IN" THAT'S NEW?

A number of years ago, Dr. James H. Cyriax[1], an English physician (and more recently, Robin McKenzie[2], a New Zealand physical therapist) taught that in cases where a bulging disk causes the body to tilt, one can, by positioning and squeezing the chest and pelvis, cause an apparent shift of the disk contents toward its proper central location, allowing the body to resume its normal alignment. Although thus far no one has actually been able to see this happen within the disk of a living patient, thousands of patients have experienced the reality of having their backs realigned or put "back in" by this "shift correction" method. An exercise and posture program that relies on the extended posture of the spine to keep the injured disk from bulging is then

---

[1]*Textbook of Orthopaedic Medicine, Volume Two*, James Cyriax, Bailliere Tindall, London, 1984.
[2]McKenzie, Robin A. The lumbar spine: mechanical diagnosis and therapy (Waikanae, N.Z.: Spinal Publications, 1981).

employed, with the idea of helping the healing process and preventing recurrences. Not all physicians are aware of this approach, which is called the *Extension Treatment Method*, but it is rapidly gaining acceptance.

This squeezing and positioning extension method typically works well in younger patients with gooey disks. It is a procedure that can take a few minutes to perform and thus is considerably different from the rapid thrust or abrupt twist that we associate with typical spinal manipulation methods. In middle-aged and older patients, the extension technique is less often useful, and in these older patients with drier disks and worn, osteoarthritic facet joints, the quick thrusting manipulations may occasionally be helpful in causing an abrupt restoration of spinal alignment in a back that's "gone out."

SNAP, CRACKLE, AND POP

The older disk typically contains hard dried fragments, which can be shifted out of position by back strains and which may push against the outer ring-fiber of the annulus fibrosus or actually rupture through the ring. If the latter situation occurs, back pain caused by pressure on the ring fibers may be relieved by the reduced disk pressure that occurs as the material from inside of the disk breaks out, but this will be followed by more serious sciatic pain if the disk material presses against a nerve root.

It has been demonstrated by Dr. H.F. Farfan[3] of Montreal in cadaver dissections that disk fragments can be moved within the disk by stimulated disk manipulations. No one, however, has been able to unequivocally demonstrate that disk fragments can actually be made to move within the disk space in a back pain sufferer. So we are left with the "ins": all of those patients whose backs were "out" and then, with a sudden twist, were "in" again—and the "outs": the doubters who still wait for positive proof that manipulation (by osteopaths, chiropractors, manual therapists, and some M.D.s) "works." Perhaps our rapidly advancing technology will give us the answers before too long!

But the "in-out" story does not end here. There is a large school of thought that places the "in-out" problem in the small spinal facet joints or in the large sacroiliac joints. It was argued

[3]*Mechanical Disorders of the Low Back*, H.F. Farfan, Lea & Febiger, Philadelphia, 1973.

for a long time that sacroiliac joints do not move and therefore could not "go out," but this has been clearly shown to be wrong. The joints do move slightly. However, detecting any change in their alignment—in, out, or "just right"—is so difficult that no convincing studies have yet been reported that prove either that sacroiliac joint displacements play any role in causing back pain or that manipulation designed to "correct" malalignments of the sacroiliac joints makes any difference in the outcome or recovery from back pain.

The small facet joints are another story. These joints lie on either side of the spinous processes—the "back bones" that you feel along the middle of your back (see pg. 9; Fig. 4). They are true joints, just like those between the bones in your fingers. Since they connect a vertebra below to the one above, these joints guide spinal motion as the spine bends and twists around the disks. When a disk is compressed, twisted, or bent, the facet joints that lie just behind this disk are also moved and may be strained. For some strange reason, the last facet joints, L5-S1 (the lumbosacral joint—between the fifth or last lumbar vertebra and the top of the sacrum), frequently develop at awkward angles and are particularly susceptible to injury.

Facet joints, like other joints in the body, are also susceptible to wear-and-tear changes, which lead to degenerative or so-called osteoarthritis (see pg. 110). In this osteoarthritic joint disorder, the facet joint surface, which is normally composed of smooth cartilage, is worn thin, and extra bone is formed at the edge of the joint. The joint loses its smooth surface and becomes irregular. A forceful movement of the body may then be transmitted through the disk, causing the facet joint on one side to gap and on the opposite side to pinch. If the joint surfaces are irregular, or if a fold of the joint lining gets pinched, the joint may become painfully stuck or "locked." The patient may lean either toward the pinched side, as a consequence of the locked movement, or to the opposite side and forward as his body attempts to move away from the painful joint.

Although there is no proof, it is thought that a manipulative thrust or a sudden spontaneous twist (turning in bed)—so quick that the strong protective contraction of the spinal muscles is taken off guard and they remain relaxed—allows the facet joints (and the associated disk) to be jarred open and gapped so that these joints release any joint lining that has been pinched. The freed joints can once again slide back into their customary alignment. This rapid reopening of the joint can cause an audible cracking sound, which is most impressive. The crack, however, may occur from the abrupt opening distraction of any nearby joint—witness the distracting sounds made by our nervous friends who habitually crack their knuckles—and does not necessarily mean that the affected facet joint or disk has been readjusted and "fixed." Nonetheless, many of us learn to do, or have a professional perform, a jerking or twisting movement that causes a "satisfying" cracking sound and seems to provide relief from pain and tension in the muscles and joints of the neck and back—or indeed, of the knuckles if you are a "knuckle cracker."

MANIPULATION AS A TREATMENT—
TRICK OR TREAT?

Why is spinal manipulation so controversial? First and foremost, from a scientific standpoint, there is no proof that manipulation does what it is said to do. Recent studies have shown that manipulation of the lumbar spine for low back pain does not improve the final outcome. In other words, patients do not get any better in the sense that their backs are somehow spared from further trouble because they have been manipulated. But manipulation has, in several studies, been shown to shorten the duration of pain and of the concomitant disability. This is not an inconsiderable benefit if one considers the alternative, the cost of more prolonged therapy, the loss of wages, and the duration of misery that can potentially be shortened.

So even if we do not know precisely how manipulation works but if it appears it may help—*why are doctors reluctant to do it? Primum non nocere:* First, do no harm. That is the first law of medicine. Since manipulation is far from consistent in its results, and since most back problems can be treated successfully without manipulation, manipulation for back pain must be used judiciously. Since manipulation can cause pain; can cause a bulging disk to rupture, aggravating or causing a sciatic nerve problem; and can cause a fracture of fragile bones in patients with bone disease, it stands to reason that reliance on manipulation as the first line of treatment for back pain sufferers is ill advised. Nonetheless, where a careful examination excludes causes other than a disk problem (bone tumor, infection, fracture), and particularly in the absence of a pinched sciatic nerve, one or two attempts at manipulation of the low back by a skilled manual therapist (physician, osteopath, chiropractor, or physical therapist) may shorten the episode of low back pain. Manipulation, however, may aggravate your symptoms, or worse, delay proper medical treatment.

But even in cases where there has been an apparently successful manipulation, and particularly in those where it was not, the lessons illustrated in this book about proper body mechanics and therapeutic and reconditioning exercises remain of the utmost importance in the total management of low back pain, if injured disks are to heal properly, minimizing recurrences of back pain and assuring a return to normal activities.

15.

THERAPIES

AND

MEDICATIONS

One of the oldest and most controversial of therapeutic approaches to low back pain, namely manipulative therapy, has been discussed in the preceding chapter. There are many other treatments that we must now consider. The treatment most relevant to your back pain condition can be chosen with greater precision through your understanding of the nature of the treatments discussed in this chapter, their effects and side effects, and how and when they might apply to you.

RELAXATION

No matter what is going on in your life—unless perhaps you are in a fight or a race—relaxation can't hurt. By the same token, if you *feel* tense, your muscles *are* tense, and in muscles tensed by pain, the pain is in*tens*ified. Not only does tension make you more aware of pain and cause more painful muscle tension and spasm, but you are more apt to move in a jerky, stressful manner, or twist, bend, or stoop abruptly when it is not necessary. The message from your body tells you to try and relieve some of your painful muscle tension by taking a relaxation pause. The basic idea is that brief periods of relaxation, like sleep at night, are restorative. They help your brain and body "batteries" to recharge, so that the circuits can work normally, and the short circuits of pain—muscle spasm—can be interrupted.

RELAXATION METHODS

There are a number of techniques that utilize autosuggestion or what amounts to self-hypnosis, by which one can clear the mind of its daily "trash" accumulation. By thinking of nothing, or about something neutral, like the number one, or a mantra (an arbitrary word that is repeated over and over); or by focusing on a pleasant, relaxing experience—lying on the beach at the seashore—you can achieve a relaxed state. Typically, this relaxation state is more readily obtained by deliberate deep breathing and by concentrating on each inhalation and exhalation. The muscles in the jaw, scalp, hands, neck, back, legs, and feet are then consciously let go, one by one, and relaxed. With practice (and there are a number of books and audio tapes to help you practice), you can become relaxed in a few minutes, but it usually takes about 10 to 20 minutes, and relaxation cannot be forced—so if you want to relax tense back muscles, you have to "back down."

■ *Biofeedback*. Biofeedback means that you are getting information about your body (*bio*) through an instrument that records biological functions. Examples of biological functions are: the warmth of your skin (measured with a thermometer) and the tension in your muscles (detected by electrical impulses from contracting muscles). The *feedback* is a sound that gets more high pitched as the temperature rises or as your muscles tense, and lower as the temperature falls or your muscles relax. Visual displays such as dials or changing colors are also used. Biofeedback is a patient-relaxation teaching tool and should only be necessary on a weekly basis for up to eight weeks. Not everyone can respond to biofeedback, and the older we are, the more difficult it is to utilize. Biofeedback and relaxation methods are not terribly helpful for most low back pain problems and actually find their greatest application in the treatment of neck and upper back pain, tension headaches, and migraine.

Tension is a symptom of poor adjustment to stress, and your decision may be to seek professional assistance so that you can better cope with your stress. What needs to be learned is how to relax and how to take advantage of free moments to reduce tension and refresh the body (including your back) and the mind.

RELAXATION MEDICATIONS BY PRESCRIPTION

Not everyone can learn to relax quickly enough or well enough to control his/her pain. Medication can help. Sedatives and muscle relaxants tend to be overused, and antidepressants are probably not used often enough.

■ *Sedatives* (sleeping pills or tranquilizers). Commonly used sedatives are Valium, Librium, and phenobarbital. If you have severe pain and cannot sleep, you probably need something for pain (*see* "*Analgesics*," *below*). Chronic use of sedatives leads to habituation and often to increased depression. If you have moderate to minimal pain, a hot tub (if you can get in and out of it comfortably) and a glass of wine (after you get out) should help you get to sleep. If all else fails, check with your physician and use as mild a sedative as possible, and use it as sparingly as possible.

■ *Muscle Relaxants*. Muscle relaxants are closely related to tranquilizers, and in most patients they do cause sedation. Some of the common muscle relaxants are Soma and Soma Compound, Parafon and Parafon Forte, and Flexeril. Like tranquilizers, these medications do help you and your muscles to relax and may add a measure of comfort, but their use over long periods of time is best avoided.

■ *Narcotic and Nonnarcotic Analgesics* (pain relievers). Nonnarcotic analgesics are primarily over-the-counter drugs and include aspirin, acetaminophen (Tylenol), and ibuprofen (Advil). No drug is perfectly safe for everyone. If these drugs are taken according to directions on the bottle or as recommended by your doctor, and they give you relief, they are probably safe to use when you need them. Check with your doctor.

Narcotics (Darvon, Darvocet, Talwin, Percodan, Percocet, codeine, Tylenol with Codeine, etc.) are the most commonly prescribed narcotic analgesics. They are all capable of causing nausea and vomiting, constipation, difficulty urinating, drowsiness, and confusion. They are all potentially addictive. Use only as prescribed. Use as little as necessary to get relief, and use for as short a period of time as possible. It is rare for patients with low back pain at The Arthritis & Back Pain Center, who follow the directions that are provided in this book, to require narcotics for more than a few days.

■ NSAIDs (nonsteroidal anti-inflammatory, or non-aspirin, non-cortisone pain, anti-pain, and anti-inflammation drugs). These drugs include Clinoril, Feldene, Indocin, Motrin, Naprosyn, Rufen, Disalcid, and Trilisate. If used in recommended doses they are effective in many patients with arthritis. Although low back pain patients past 40 to 50 years of age typically have some "arthritic" wear-and-tear changes in the spine and facet joints, these drugs rarely are more helpful for pain control than nonnarcotic analgesics, and they don't cure the arthritis.

■ *Antidepressants.* Pain is a depressing experience. Pain can impair sleep. Both of these adverse phenomena, as well as the pain itself, can be offset to some extent by one of several drugs originally developed to treat depression and now found to be of value for treating pain. Typically, these antidepressant medications, when used to treat back pain, are used in doses less than half of that required to treat true depressive disorders. But they can cause very disturbing problems, including severe drowsiness, nightmares, difficulty urinating, constipation, dry mouth, and blurred vision. If the drugs are effective for pain control and they cause no disturbing side effects, they are sometimes used over a period of months.

OVER THE COUNTER AND THROUGH THE WOODS

A lot of bucks for very little bang may be what you get with over the counter medications. If you want aspirin you can buy Arthritis Pain Formula, Bayer Aspirin, Bufferin, Emperin, Measurin, or Ecotrin. The latter has the advantage of being coated so that the aspirin is less apt to be irritating to the stomach lining, but it is still aspirin. If you want acetaminophen, there is Tylenol, Anacin (Anacin also has a teacup of caffeine in every tablet), Datril, Phenaphen, and Percogesic. Another compound, called Parafon Forte, also has acetaminophen as an essential ingredient.

Another weak aspirinlike salicylate is New Formula Doan's pills with magnesium salicylate. If you really want to get exotic, you can still find "De Witt's pills for backache and joint pains." The De Witt's pill package has a warning, "Note: A few pills will turn the urine blue or green because of the methylene blue ingredients." That is in addition to potassium, nitrate, caffeine, and get this, Uva Ursi and Buchu (the latter two were recently removed from Doan's pills), as well as another aspirinlike substance called salicylamide, the only active ingredient. Shades of 1900!

How about a nice medicated back rub? What would you like? A little methyl salicylate, menthol, camphor, and alcohol—try Ben-Gay Clear Gel or Deep Down. For the same, minus alcohol, try Absorbine Arthritic Pain Lotion, Deep Heating Rub, Icy Hot, or Banalg. Heet gives you the methyl salicylate with alcohol and camphor instead of menthol, while Absorbine Jr. gives you methyl salicylate, menthol, and a dash of chloroxylenol. You can also get triethanolamine or trolamine salicylate if you buy certain preparations of either Aspercreme, Myoflex, or Exocaine. There are many variations on these themes—so you pays your money and you takes your choice! If you don't get a rash—it may be soothing. If you like to rub—shop before you buy, at least then the price won't rub you wrong.

THERAPIES: SOME SIMPLE, SOME DECEPTIVELY SIMPLE, SOME COMPLEX

By and large, most of us do not like to take medicines. We worry about side effects, about getting into pill popping habits, and just generally would prefer not to have to take them. Here are some alternative suggestions.

ICE MASSAGE

Cold numbs nerves that send painful messages. The use of ice massage for 2 to 3 minutes every hour, at least four times a day, over very tender spots or "trigger points" is an effective pain reliever. Freeze water in a small paper cup to make a handy applicator. A tongue blade or popsicle stick can give you a longer reach, but it's usually best if someone else applies the ice. Massage gently with firm strokes until the area is numb, and continue for 1 more minute. Prolonged ice application can produce frostbite. Too much of a good thing can be bad.

MASSAGE

Stroking massage makes almost anyone relax and feel good. Deep vigorous kneading massage can damage previously injured tissue and is to be avoided in severe or moderate levels of low back pain. Deep massage pressure over a painful trigger point (acupressure or shiatsu) for 5 to 10 seconds can sometimes lessen painful local muscle spasms in both moderate and mild cases. These types of massage are best left to experts, physical therapists, or masseurs recommended by your physician or physical therapist. Massage by a misguided or inept masseur can injure tissues and aggravate back pain problems. If you're not sure about your masseur, back off. If you're desperate to try, insist on a gentle stroking type of massage.

LINIMENTS

Liniments cause warming of the skin and can be soothing "counter-irritants." Their most common ingredient, methyl salicylate, can be absorbed through the skin. Liniments can cause blistering and are especially apt to do so if they are used with a heating pad.

HOT PACKS

Although generally less effective than cold in relieving moderate and severe skeletal pain (pain severity is a very subjective and relative thing), warm applications for moderate pain can often be soothing and help relax muscle spasm. A heating pad is usually least effective but easiest to use. A Hydrocollator heat-retaining pad or a Thermaphor moisture-attracting electric warmer pad can also be relatively easily applied. Never use a hot pack for more than 20 minutes out of each hour, and never fall asleep with a heating pad—you don't need a burn *and* back pain! A hot tub and/or Jacuzzi is also soothing, but getting in and out requires care if strain or reinjury is to be avoided.

CORSETS AND BRACES

In order to be up and about with moderate low back pain or sciatica, and especially to be able to perform tasks where the back cannot be reliably protected, a corset or brace is mandatory. It should be kept available and worn when extra back protection is required, e.g., for unavoidable household or work tasks, or during travel.

■ *Corsets.* The best all around corset is made of heavy canvas, is snapped or zippered in front, and has three straps on each side that can be cinched upward from below for a snug abdominal compression, and buttock-hugging, low-back-bracing support. Firm stays (the semi-rigid metal bands that are attached to your corset), bent to conform to your low back and buttocks, provide added support and help restrict *but do not prevent* lumbar motion. These corsets, not exactly attractive, are made in various designs to make them somewhat more appealing for women. Never accept a corset that is uncomfortable unless it has been okayed by your physician, and never take a corset out of a shop until you have been instructed and *are able* to demonstrate that you know how to put it on and take it off without straining your back.

An elastic corset is the easiest to fit and is easiest to put on. The elastic is cinched in front and held in place by Velcro and, typically, two additional overlapping straps. A firm plastic pad, custom molded against the lumbar spine and inserted in a pocket at the rear of some corsets, provides additional firmness and support. Large or obese men and women are often unable to get sufficient back support with an elastic corset, and for these people it is difficult at best with any other garment.

■ *Back Braces.* Braces may be the answer if you are heavily built and do heavy work, or if you require a brace to hold you in a special flexed posture. Back braces are generally heavy and are usually more difficult to fit than a corset. They do allow for more air circulation and are cooler and more comfortable in hot weather. Rigid plastic braces, lighter than metal framed braces, are now available, but they require careful fitting and the plastic occasionally causes a rash.

SPRAY AND STRETCH

A vapo-coolant spray is a form of hyperstimulation analgesia (see discussion below, under TNS). A gentle spray with *fluorimethane* (a highly volatile substance that cools by rapid evaporation) along the muscle with a trigger area in spasm is repeated slowly in several passes. The tense muscle relaxes and is gently stretched. The key appears to be the induction of temporary muscle relaxation by cooling, which permits a good muscle stretch and an interruption of the pain-spasm cycle. This requires assistance because you can't twist around to spray many of the muscles that may need it. A physician or therapist can teach a family member or friend the proper techniques for spraying and stretching if you have recurrent muscle spasms that respond to this method of treatment.

TRANSCUTANEOUS NERVE STIMULATION (TNS)

Transcutaneous nerve stimulation (TNS or TENS) is a form of what is called *hyperstimulation analgesia*. It is now thought that a variety of strong (although not necessarily painful) stimuli, such as the electrical currents used in TNS, or such as acupuncture, acupressure, vibration, massage, cold or ice massage, rubbing a bruise, or the traditional "biting the bullet," act at least in part by a similar mechanism that is the result of a strong stimulation (*hyperstimulation*) to the nerves. TNS is administered by passing an electric current from a card-deck-sized battery-powered current-generating device, attached to a belt or bra, through electrodes taped to the skin. This sends a message along these nerves to the spinal cord, and to the brain nerve centers, that causes the body to liberate its own morphinelike pain blockers called *endorphins*. Although not always effective, these TNS devices must be prescribed by a physician and can be rented or purchased from a medical or surgical supply company for use at home or at work. TNS often permits control of pain that might otherwise require narcotics or surgery for relief.

TNS is also administered by passing a smaller current through a blunt metal probe placed on the skin overlying painful areas.

These devices, called *point stimulators* or *neuroprobes*, are applied where nerves emerge just under the skin and permit easy transmission of smaller currents. Point stimulation takes less time than ordinary TNS. It is more often associated with discomfort during or following treatment, but it often relieves pain for hours to days.

Skin irritation as well as discomfort can be brought on by these devices. Patients with cardiac pacemakers, metal plates, or artificial joints in their bodies, or those who are pregnant, may have more serious problems due to electrical short circuiting, and the use of a TNS is not advised in such patients.

ACUPUNCTURE

Acupuncture is a system of medical treatment by means of fine needle insertion into specified acupuncture points and is used for essentially all illness. It originated in China and is widely used all over Asia for a variety of purposes, including pain control. With the renewal of our trade with China, acupuncture was rediscovered in the West, but almost exclusively for use as a pain control measure. There is evidence that acupuncture works in part by stimulating the body to produce endorphins (see TNS, above).

Pain is complex, our knowledge of the chemistry and physiology of pain is still rudimentary, and the techniques used by acupuncturists are quite variable and often seem arbitrary to Western-trained physicians (although many trigger points coincide with acupuncture points). However, there are now a respectable number of research studies to support the claims that acupuncture can control many kinds of pain at least temporarily—for hours to days. Acupuncture is quite safe, relatively costly, and typically requires visits twice weekly to a licensed acupuncturist. In this day of concern for AIDS, the use of disposable needles is a basic safety precaution.

ACUPRESSURE

Acupressure (shiatsu) is the use of deep pressure instead of needles over painful tender and nontender acupuncture points. This, too, is safe if done by a trained therapist, and it can, with proper instruction, be learned for use as a self-administered pain control measure.

DIATHERMY AND ULTRASOUND

Diathermy and ultrasound were once thought to be cure-alls for painful disorders. Today diathermy (it means deep heat) is hardly used, and ultrasound is no longer felt to be dependably effective—especially for relatively severe low back pain.

Diathermy works by either electromagnetic radiation or microwaves, (the most commonly used form heats like your microwave oven). Ultrasound is another method of deep heating which uses a sound wave pitched beyond our hearing ability, hence *ultra*sound. Ultrasound can penetrate deep into muscles and ligaments and heat them. This deep heat can relieve pain and promote healing in some cases with chronic areas of strain, but usually it is not strikingly helpful, and moreover, not infrequently it will aggravate severe pain.

TRACTION

Spinal traction is a method used to stretch the spine. Traction probably works primarily by stretching tight muscles and overcoming painful muscle spasm. When the muscles are stretched, the underlying disks, nerves, and facet joints may be placed under a reduced strain and therefore become less painful. It is generally assumed that malaligned disk fragments or facet joints can cause pain (*see "Snap, Crackle, and Pop," pg. 122*) and that this is eased by restoring the disks or facet joints to a more normal structural alignment when the compressive forces of body weight and muscle spasm are relieved through traction. It can be done with the patient in bed, by means of a girdle that is attached by ropes over pulleys to weights that hang over the end of the bed; or by hanging upright from a horizontal bar or from the top of a door (not too comfortable), or hanging suspended vertically either right-side-up, or more popularly, upside-down. It takes a force of about one half of your body weight to get any separation between the lumbar vertebrae. Therefore, most traction done in a hospital with between 20 and 40 pounds of weight attached to a sling around your pelvis does nothing as far as stretching the spine is concerned. It does keep you quietly in bed—not necessarily a bad thing, but really not an effective use of traction per se.

There is no persuasive evidence that traction can suck protruding disks back into place—no matter how much force is applied. In fact, when the compression force of the body weight on the disks is relieved by traction, the disk can actually absorb more water than when it is compressed and thereby become swollen. This probably accounts for the not uncommon aggravation of symptoms after a traction treatment.

■ *The Safest Traction*—Horizontal traction on specially designed friction-free tables permits precisely controlled traction that can be tailored to a patient's needs and tolerance. Patients can readily get on and off a traction table, and they can rest there after a treatment. Used once-or-twice-daily or every-other-day for about 20 minutes, with an effective disk-separating force of about 50% of the body weight, horizontal traction can relieve moderate to severe lumbar disk pain and/or sciatic pressure. When traction is helpful, the pain is partially relieved for hours to days after the brief traction session, and traction usually needs to be repeated daily or every other day for one to two weeks for maximum benefit. Traction is always part of a total treatment program and is never relied upon as *the* treatment.

■ *Vertical Traction—Upright.* Aside from patients who find grasping the top of a door and hanging to be helpful, the major advocates of vertical upright traction have been the Kenny Institute physicians in Minneapolis. This treatment program typically requires hospitalization at first and up to months of daily suspension in a special harness on a tilting table that allows the patient to "hang" upright. Whether this demanding treatment has anything unique to offer over and above other treatment methods or other forms of traction remains to be proved.

■ *Vertical Traction—Inverted.* Let it all hang out!

This is no longer the current rage. It is not a cure-all and it is not trouble-free. The idea is the same as that of any other traction—to unload the spine and take pressure off the disks. The method has inspired some creative advertising copy, but there is no convincing data to support the claims of its supposed benefits.

At The Arthritis & Back Pain Center, we have found very few patients who benefit from any of the several types of inverted traction devices we have been evaluating. Many patients have difficulty getting on or off these devices, which are to be avoided by the weak or poorly coordinated among us. Those devices that require boots can cause ankle pain, and getting in and out of the boots can strain your back. Those that require leaning over leg pads can cause severe thigh pain. Hanging upside down raises the blood pressure, stresses the heart, and causes potentially dangerous congestion in the eyes. Exercises while hanging can be injurious—so hang around a little before you jump in and flip out or—let it hang out!

In our experience, the rare patients who have benefited sufficiently to continue using inverted traction, for typically 2 to 5 minutes once or twice a day, are patients with chronic mild back discomfort who experience increased aching at the end of the day, or after unusual activity or prolonged inactivity. The stretch on the hanging traction device seems to relax their muscles and (perhaps equally important) relax them psychologically.

SPECIAL INJECTION PROCEDURES

TRIGGER POINT AND TENDER JOINT INJECTIONS

Trigger point and tender point injections are often helpful in relieving persistent areas of aching, tenderness, and pain that accompanies movement in the low back, buttocks, or thighs. When the tender point is caused by a small knot of muscle spasm, an injection of a local anesthetic, like Novocain, will often block the nerve to the muscle and relax the spasm. This relaxation of the spasm persists long after the anesthetic effort has worn off. In fact, one such anesthetic injection may, by stopping a "short circuited" reflex (spinal cord stimulation—muscle spasm—pain in muscle), give prolonged and even permanent relief from a painful trigger point.

Tender point irritation and irritation in the bursae (bursitis) in the buttocks and hips are also responsive to injections, into the tender areas, of small, safe amounts of cortisone-like steroid (often about what your own adrenal glands make each day), usually combined with a local anesthetic. This cortisone-anesthetic mixture is frequently used in trigger points as well, but in my experience, the addition of cortisone to muscle trigger point injections rarely adds any great benefit.

FACET JOINT INJECTIONS

Persistent back pain localized to one of the facet joints can, like a painful knee or tennis elbow, sometimes be relieved by a cortisone-like injection into the joint. The exact location of the joint is determined by the use of an X-ray fluoroscope. Typically, the joint is first numbed with a local anesthetic (Novocain) to relieve the pain and to confirm that the suspected joint is the source of the pain. A small amount of cortisone-like medication is then injected into the joint. This procedure is technically somewhat difficult, but no more dangerous than injecting any other joint. Facet joint injections are done in physicians' offices or as a hospital outpatient procedure, and the patient can go home under his/her own power shortly after the injection is done.

EPIDURAL STEROID INJECTIONS

A moderate amount of cortisone-like (steroid) drug is injected into the spinal canal, either by a *lumbar puncture* (the needle is inserted between the vertebral spines from behind) or by a *caudal injection* (the needle is inserted through a small opening on the sacrum at the bottom of your pelvis, just above the tailbone, and is pushed on into the spinal canal). In the presence of a disk-related sciatic nerve irritation that is judged not to be improving, there is about a 50% chance that the healing process will be enhanced and the pain will be relieved with the aid of epidural steroid injections. Typically, if these injections are going to help, one to three injections suffice. Rarely, a fourth or more injections can be of additional value. Epidural steroid injections can be done in a specialist's office or as a hospital outpatient procedure, usually once or twice a week. They do require a physician's supervision and follow-up because of the possibility of spinal nerve injury, and because the amount of the cortisone-like drug that is injected is significant and cortisone side effects must be monitored.

16.

SURGERY—

THE CUTTING

EDGE

If your back pain problem defies all reasonable efforts at treatment, gets steadily worse despite treatment, or doesn't improve enough to let you get on with your life on terms that are acceptable to you, you are facing a tough decision. You should have a physician helping you, and now may be the time for a second opinion, because you are possibly talking about an operation.

What are the surgical options?

A STEP BACK FROM SURGERY—
CHEMONUCLEOLYSIS

An enzyme called *chymopapain* (the same substance found in papaya and used as a meat tenderizer) can dissolve the nucleus of the disk. It has to be injected from the back, into the bulging disk, with a long needle. This is done by a surgeon in the hospital under X-ray visualization, usually with the patient asleep under a general anesthetic. When there is only back pain, you probably don't need this. When the disk is worn down and dried out, it won't work. When the annulus has torn so that the disk contents of the nucleus are now in the spinal canal and pressing on nerve roots, it's too late. But if you have an intact bulging disk (remember, there is about a 10 to 20% chance of error with all of the diagnostic tests) causing spinal nerve pressure and severe or moderate symptoms, then there is about a 75% chance that you will benefit from chemonucleolysis and can avoid surgery. If your symptoms are only mild, your chance of benefit is much less because you have less to gain.

It's important to know that this procedure can only be done once, because of the risk of a subsequent serious allergic reaction after this foreign material has once been put in your body. The risks of chemonucleolysis are death from the anesthetic (the same risk as an appendectomy) and severe allergic reactions (to the chymopapain). Several cases of permanent paralysis from chymopapain have been reported. This procedure was banned in the United States for several years because of a few patients' severe allergic reactions to chymopapain and because of failure to prove its effectiveness. You can expect up to a month of severe backache brought about by irritation in the disk as a result of the enzyme injection.

Keep in mind that if your problem is a backache due to a bulging disk without nerve root pressure, it will likely get well in a month anyway with proper treatment and no chymopapain. Also, there is a rare possibility for infection (*osteomyelitis*) to occur in the treated disk space. Lastly, we do know that you will stand a little less tall when your disk has been enzymatically shrunken, but we really do not know how many patients are going to develop severe osteoarthritis in their facet joints as a result of increased wear and tear after the shock absorbing disk has been dissolved.

NO-WAY-BACK SURGERY!

If a persistent disk bulge keeps you in the severe or moderate pain category (*see Table 1, "Pain Levels at a Glance," pg. 43*) with or without nerve root pressure, and chemonucleolysis either failed or was not deemed advisable by your surgeon, you're going to need an operation.

GOOD NEWS FOR BAD BACKS—SURGERY

■ *Microsurgery.* In the last few years, as a consequence of the success of operating through an arthroscope into the knee and other joints, a similar technique has been developed for operating on disk problems. In the situations where chemonucleolysis has proven to be most useful, namely a small discrete disk bulge that's pressing on a branch of the sciatic nerve, the development of microsurgery offers an attractive alternative. In fact, recent studies comparing microsurgery to chemonucleolysis have shown an advantage for microsurgery: fewer complications, shorter hospital stay, less postoperative discomfort, and overall better results.

■ *Percutaneous diskectomy.* Percutaneous diskectomy is the latest wrinkle in disk surgery. The procedure consists of placing a long, large-bore needle through the back muscles on one side of the spine right into the center of the disk. A tiny blade is passed through the needle into the center of the disk, and this cutting blade is whirled at a high speed to mince the inner disk tissues, similar to the action of a blender. A mild salt solution flows down through the needle and helps to liquify the chopped disk material. This material is then aspirated out of the body by suction through an inner tube within the needle. The result is the creation of a hole within the disk similar to that which occurs when the disk is dissolved by chemonucleolysis. The bulging disk material can then collapse back in toward the center of the disk, removing pressure on the annulus and/or sciatic nerves. The advantage of this procedure is that it can be done under local anesthetic and does not require the introduction of a foreign substance (chymopapain), which can cause allergic reactions. Its disadvantage is that the cutting procedure is done "blindly": the surgeon cannot see the delicate nerves and other structures that might inadvertently be damaged. This new technique may well prove to have a useful place in the treatment of small disk bulges and to present an alternative in such cases to microsurgery.

LAMINOTOMY, THE CONVENTIONAL DISK OPERATION

Prior to the advent of microsurgery, the laminotomy was considered the most conservative operative technique. In this operation, the surgeon attempts to remove as small a piece of bone overlying the spinal canal as possible, so that he can see the extent of the disk protrusion and avoid injury to the delicate spinal nerves. The name laminotomy comes from the word *lamina* (the table of bone overlying the spinal cord and nerves) and *otomy* (the hole that is made in that bony table). Once the protruding disk material is visualized, the surgeon then scrapes it out and you are sewed back up. The laminotomy is the procedure of choice when the disk bulge is a large one or when an attempt at chemonucleolysis or microsurgery has failed and a more extensive procedure is required. In any event, if you survive the operation, if there are no complications, if the correct disk bulge was removed, and if you had moderate or severe sciatica and not just back pain before surgery, then there is a 90% chance of a good outcome.

There may also be a painfully poor outcome if the diagnosis was incorrect, if surgery damaged delicate nerve tissue or the small facet joints, or if excessive scar tissue forms after surgery, causing the nerve root to become stuck and tethered to adjacent structures in the spine. If your surgery was performed to relieve numbness or paralysis, rather than for sciatic pain per se, the chances for a good outcome are only about 50:50 and the possibilities for complications are of course still there.

LAMINECTOMY

When there is a large protrusion, or when spinal stenosis is present, a larger incision is mandatory and the entire lamina may need to be removed (*laminectomy*). This used to be a fairly routine procedure, but because there is more tissue destruction and therefore more chance for complications, the more limited laminotomy is done whenever feasible.

SPINAL FUSION

This is a very major operation. One technique consists of putting a bone plug, like a dowel, upright between the fronts of two of the vertebral bodies to cause them to stick together. It sounds simple but actually is a very dangerous procedure because of the possibility of injuring the major blood vessels that lie just in front of the vertebrae. A more common procedure consists of the application of struts of bone taken from the pelvis (iliac bone) and chips taken from the spine. They are inserted into channels made on either side of the denuded bone overlying the spinal canal. This bone graft almost always includes the sacrum and the fifth lumbar vertebra, and may go higher in certain cases. The hope is that these bone chips and struts will all fuse and prevent further painful motion of the spine. Casting and bracing for many months are mandatory to prevent any motion that could interfere with a solid fusion—but even so, a solid fusion is only achieved about half of the time. Because this is such a big operation, there are many more opportunities for things to go wrong, and they often do. Nonetheless, with a severe spondylolisthesis or unrelenting facet osteoarthritis, or in a patient with deforming *scoliosis* (twisting spine), spinal fusion may offer the only hope for restoration to relatively normal, comfortable function.

BACK AGAIN OR STILL BACK THERE?

What if you've had surgery and you're not better, or are worse off? If you've not really had a good conservative program, such as is outlined in this book, there is an excellent chance that, with such a program, you'll be able to improve—you can get on the road back! If you have had back surgery, or if you have been advised not to, but have had the opportunity to follow a well supervised program of back care, and you are still miserable, you may need to learn to live with it. Wait—that's not a statement of no help. You can learn to live and enjoy life even with pain. Pain Centers have sprung up all over the country. Many are not much better than quack factories—but some, particularly at or affiliated with a university medical center, provide a useful variety of treatments, with heavy emphasis on teaching self-control of pain. This is done by means of self-hypnosis; by learning not to make pain the focus of your life; by intensive reconditioning exercises, and by group activities and therapy where you see others like yourself learning to cope effectively. Don't let pain be your justification for losing. In the game of life, there are many ways to play. Find ways to win. Engage in activities that involve your mind and your spirit so your *low back pain* just becomes a *low pain* in the *back*. Don't be shackled by your pain—rather, let it be a spur to fulfilling life.

IV.

ERGONOMICS:

BACK PAIN

PROTECTION AND

PREVENTION

17.

BACK PROTECTION

PRINCIPLES

AND FUNDAMENTALS

A PENNY SAVED

A penny saved is a penny earned. A back pain saved is worth thousands. The total annual cost of back pain in this country is now at twenty billion dollars per year. Now, that's a stack of thousand dollar bills about fifty stories high! That's real money!

Obviously it pays to save your back. There's no fair price or even a market rate on your pain and suffering, but you know that the cost is dear. It clearly pays to pay attention to the details in the nitty gritty of daily activity that might have an adverse effect on your back—or better, that might permit you to do something in a way that would otherwise be painfully impossible.

Ergonomics is the term we have used to refer to the efficiency and economy with which we function in different environments and at different tasks (*ergo* meaning work and *nomics* meaning economically). Ergonomics addresses the relationship between people and the environment. It concentrates on the design of products, as well as the arrangement of the environment, so that they are adapted to the user rather than vice versa. Ergonomics is concerned with the comfort and satisfaction of people at work and at play. The Arthritis & Back Pain Center's Back Protection Ergonomics described in this chapter are basic guides to preventive care for your back. Presented in eight basic instruction sheets, these carefully worded handouts have proven extremely useful in instructing our back pain patients at the Center, and will be helpful to you as well. Read them carefully, learn them well, practice them faithfully, and you will make a large investment in your back savings account.

BACK PROTECTION PRINCIPLES
(BACK PROTECTION ERGONOMICS)

#1 BACK FIRST—BACK FLAT—BACK STRAIGHT—BACK LAST *(the Four Back Words)*

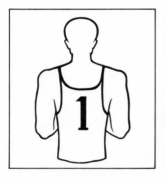

BACK FIRST
HOW?
Plan ahead and think of *back protection first!*

WHEN?
Organizing each day and your daily activities—avoid fatigue and strain from activity that is *too* strenuous, *too* hurried, or *too* erratic.

Lying or sitting
Select furniture that is supportive. For example: a firm mattress and chairs with back support. (*See Chapter 18, "Take a Back Seat," and Chapter 19, "Back in Bed."*)

Lifting, carrying, or reaching
To carry heavy objects, use a cart on wheels. To pick up objects from the floor, squat down. To reach objects from above your head, use a footstool or a stepladder. Use a long-handled reaching-stick when objects cannot be easily grasped from the floor or overhead.

Dressing
To put on your shoes, use a long-handled shoe horn to avoid

bending forward at the waist; or sit down and bring your foot up to you.

BACK FLAT
HOW?
Perform a mild pelvic tilt (pinch buttocks together and tighten stomach muscles (*see Exercise #1, pg. 225*) before initiating any movement. This will help maintain spinal alignment.

WHEN?

Lying
Bend your knees to maintain the "back flat" posture. On your back, have a pillow under your knees. On your side, place a pillow between the knees.

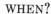

Sitting
Keep your knees higher than your waist or at the same level as your hips by using a footstool.

Standing
Bend one knee by placing your foot on a stool or rail. Support your back in a mild pelvic tilt against the wall whenever possible.

BACK STRAIGHT
HOW?
If possible, move your torso as one unit.

WHEN?

Lying
Keeping your knees bent, place your hands on your thighs and roll your body to turn in bed, moving your shoulders, trunk, and knees together as one unit ("log roll").

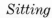

Sitting
Have a chair that provides good lumbar support and swivels, or use a small pillow in the low back to provide lumbar support (*see Chapter 18*).

Standing
To turn, pivot with feet.

FEET FIRST AND FACE IT—Whenever possible, when sitting or standing, turn your entire body as a unit, moving your feet first, in order to face your task.

PRECAUTIONS—AVOID:
Extending backwards, as in reaching too far overhead. Use a stepstool instead.
Twisting!
Bending forward at the waist.

BACK LAST
HOW?
First use your legs and arms to initiate and assist all movement.

WHEN?
Lifting
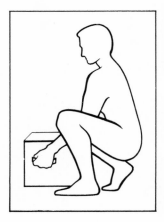
Move close to the object or slide the object close to your body; then squat or kneel before lifting.

Pushing rather than pulling
Bend your knees and position your arms close to your body.

Reaching
Use a footstool or stepladder to reach overhead objects.

#2 DOWN AND UP FROM BED

DOWN:

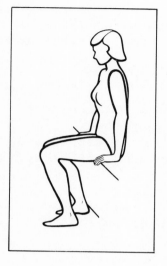

1. Feel the edge of the bed with the backs of your legs. Place your "most comfortable leg" backward under the edge of the bed (*if possible*).

2. Do a mild pelvic tilt and hold. Bend your knees to lower yourself onto the edge of the bed. Use your hands to help support you.

3. Use your arms and hands to lift your buttocks and scoot back into a comfortable seated position on the bed.

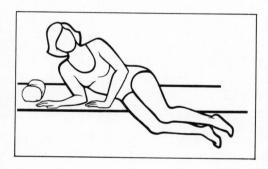

4. Place both hands on the bed *on the side toward the head of the bed.* Slide your hands toward the pillow to support your body as you gently swing your legs onto the bed (*you should now be in a side lying position*).

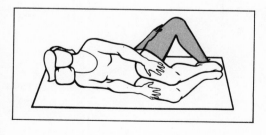

5. Keeping your knees bent, place your hands on your thighs and roll onto your back moving your shoulders, trunk, and knees together as one unit (*"log roll"*).

6. Adjust your legs one at a time for comfort.

UP:

1. Lying on your back with your knees bent, do a mild pelvic tilt and hold.

2. Holding the pelvic tilt, place your hands on your thighs and roll onto your side moving shoulders, trunk, and knees together as a unit (*"log roll"*).

3. Raise your shoulders by pushing off the bed with your hand and elbow; at the same time gently swing both legs over the side of the bed.

4. Use your arms and hands to help lift and slide your buttocks to the edge of the bed.

5. Place one foot slightly in front of the other with the rear foot (*your most comfortable leg*) under the bed (*if possible*).

6. Keeping your buttocks tucked under (pelvic tilt) and your back straight, use your arms and legs to push up to a standing position.

#3 DOWN AND UP FROM A CHAIR

DOWN:

STRAIGHT CHAIR:

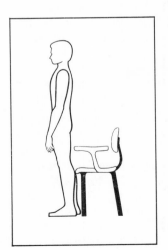

1. Feel the front of the chair with the backs of your legs. Place your "most comfortable leg" backward under the edge of the chair (*if possible*).

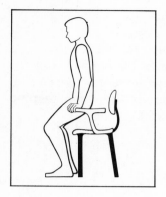

2. Do a mild pelvic tilt. While holding the pelvic tilt, bend your knees to lower yourself onto the front of the chair.

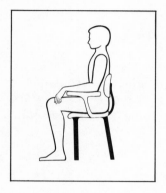

3. Using your hands to support, scoot your buttocks to the rear of the chair until your back is supported.

ARMCHAIR:

1. Feel the front of the chair with the backs of your legs. Place your "most comfortable leg" backward under the edge of the chair (*if possible*).

2. Do a mild pelvic tilt. While holding the pelvic tilt, reach down for the chair arms for support as you bend your knees to lower yourself onto the front of the chair.

3. Also use the chair arms for support to help you scoot to the rear of the seat.

UP:

STRAIGHT CHAIR OR ARMCHAIR:

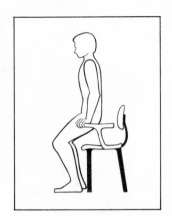

1. Using your hands for support (*on the arms of the chair or seat of the chair*), scoot to the edge of the chair keeping your back straight.

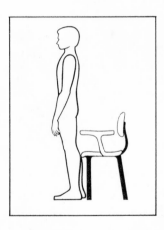

2. Place one foot slightly in front of the other with the rear foot (*most comfortable leg*) under the chair (*if possible*).

3. Keeping your buttocks tucked under (*pelvic tilt*) and your back straight, use your arms and legs to push up to a standing position.

POINTS TO REMEMBER:

1. Use a rolled towel or folded sweater, or a small pillow or purse, to support the curve of your lower back when necessary.

2. Place your knees equal to or slightly higher than your hips, and place your feet firmly on the floor or on a small footstool.

3. Choose a chair with a high firm seat, a firm back, and armrests whenever possible.

#4 HIP BENDING

BACK FIRST

1. Protect your back by using your hips and not your back.

BACK FLAT

2. Pinch your buttocks together and tighten your stomach muscles (do a mild pelvic tilt).
3. Bend your knees slightly. Support your body with your hands or elbows whenever possible.

BACK STRAIGHT

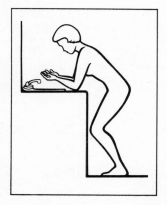

4. Keeping your knees bent, move your buttocks backwards. Your back should remain straight.

TO RETURN TO STANDING POSITION:

1. Keeping your knees bent, bring your buttocks back under you (pelvic tilt).

BACK LAST

2. Straighten your knees.

#5 SQUATTING

To put an object down or to prepare for lifting:

BACK FIRST

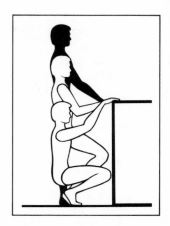

1. Face the object with your feet shoulder distance apart and with your stronger leg behind.

BACK FLAT

2. Pinch your buttocks together and tighten your stomach muscles (mild pelvic tilt). Keep your chin in and your back flat as you lower yourself by bending your knees (your hips will bend simultaneously).

BACK STRAIGHT

3. Keep your chin in and hold a mild pelvic tilt as you straighten your knees to come to a standing position.

BACK LAST

4. Remember to avoid twisting. *Feet First and Face It!*

Alternative Suggestions on Squatting.
A. Place your feet side by side (*shoulders width apart*).
B. Have one foot in front of the other with your stronger leg behind (*step position*), as described previously.
C. Place your hands on your thighs for support when squatting down and rising up.

D. For side support while squatting, hold onto a heavy table, chair, or counter with one hand. To avoid leaning forward, have the chair at your side before squatting.

E. Hold onto a cane, stick, or mop handle to provide additional support while squatting.

F. If you don't have knee problems, kneel onto one leg. If possible, place a small pillow or folded towel under your knee.

G. When possible, squat to sit on a small stool for more prolonged activities at a low level.

THINK ABOUT SQUATTING PROPERLY

In your home environment:
—making beds, doing laundry, in bathroom activities
—getting into low cupboards and other kitchen activities
—participating in garden activities

In your work environment:
—looking in file cabinets
—reaching for books or papers in low drawers

#6 DOWN AND UP FROM THE FLOOR

DOWN:

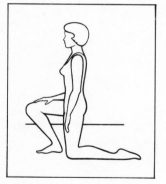

1. Stand comfortably with your feet apart. If possible, plan to use additional support with one hand on your thigh (*or a table, chair, or bed*) to help maintain your balance.

2. Slowly lower yourself onto the knee of your stronger leg while maintaining a straight back. (*If a knee or leg is painful, kneel on the more comfortable side.*)

3. Put your other knee on the floor (*kneel-ing position*) and your arms at your sides.

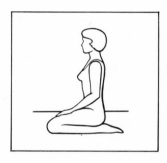

4. Place your hands on your thighs for support as you lower your buttocks down onto your heels while keeping your back straight.

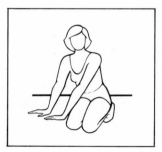

5. Lean to your comfortable side, placing both hands about a shoulders' width apart on the floor as you shift your buttocks off your heels and onto the floor. Avoid twisting!

6. Lower yourself as smoothly as possible onto your outer forearm.

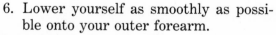

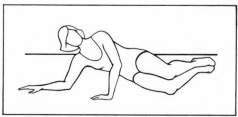

7. Continue the movement as you slide your outer elbow beneath your body. Now you will be in a side-lying position.

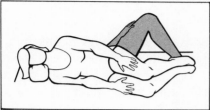

8. Keeping your knees bent, do a mild pelvic tilt. Moving your shoulders, trunk, and knees together as unit, roll onto your back (*"log roll"*).

UP:

1. Lie on your back with your knees bent; do a mild pelvic tilt.

2. Moving your shoulders, trunk, and knees together, roll onto your (*left or right*) side (*"log roll"*).

3. Keeping your back straight and using your hands for support, push up onto your outer forearm.

4. Push up onto your outer hand and continue "walking" your hands toward your knees to assist you as you shift your buttocks up onto your heels.

5. Raise up to a kneeling position with your back straight. Use additional support by placing your hands on your thighs (*or a table, chair, or bed*) if you wish.

6. Bring your strong leg forward. Place your hand on the forward knee and push up to a standing position.

#7 LIFTING

ACUTE PHASE (Severe Pain, Level 4 to Moderate Pain, Level 3)

1. In the acute phase, *do not lift!* Ask someone to lift for you.

2. If you must lift do not allow the object to exceed 5 pounds.

LIFTING OBJECTS (Moderate Pain, Level 3 to Mild Pain, Level 2)

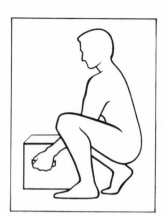

1. Keeping your chin in and maintaining a mild pelvic tilt, face the object, squat to the floor, and pick up the object. In order to take proper hold of a large object, grip it with your palms and fingers. Keep your elbows in at your sides and keep the load close to your chest. *Remember:* Avoid twisting by *pivoting* with your feet in order to face load when lifting—for both standing or squatting position. *Feet First and Face It!*

2. Keep your chin in and maintain a pelvic tilt as you straighten your knees to come to a standing position.

ALTERNATIVE SUGGESTIONS ON LIFTING
A. Lift with one hand and use the other hand for leverage (*on a counter, chair, or on your thigh*) to push off to a standing position.
B. Hold onto a heavy table, chair, or counter and go onto one knee to lift an object. Remember to tighten your buttock and stomach muscles and then bend at the hips (*see "Hip Bending," pg. 155*) to reach for the object.
C. If the object is too heavy—don't lift. Ask two or more people to help you.

SPECIAL SITUATIONS FOR LIFTING
A. *Lifting an object under a shelf or a table*
    1. Use a stick, cane, or hanger to pull objects close to you (*out from under the table*).
    2. How to lift:
        a. Face the object and get down onto your hands and knees (*maintaining a mild pelvic tilt*).
        b. Attempt to push or pull the object out.

   c. Grasp the object to your chest. Come to a kneeling position.
   d. Use your stronger leg to come up to a half kneeling (*one knee*) position.
   e. Utilize the strength in both legs to stand.
B. *Lifting an object from an intermediate height* (e.g., groceries from a basket, object from the car trunk or from a coffee table)
   1. How to lift:
      a. Face the object you are going to lift.
      b. Keep your chin in and maintain as much of a pelvic tilt as needed to keep your back from arching, then bend with your knees and then at your hips (*hip bending*).
      c. Lift the object in toward your chest.
      d. Straighten your knees and hips simultaneously.

   SUGGESTIONS
   When lifting grocery bags from a basket, use the rim of the basket as a middle step to hold the weight of the bag. In a car trunk, use the seal of the trunk as a middle step to gain support while lifting. If the object is light enough, use your free hand on your thigh for support in lifting your body and the object.

C. *Lifting heavy objects* (*do this in stages!*)
   1. Place a chair close to the object you are going to lift. *Remember:* Avoid twisting by pivoting with your feet, while standing or squatting, to face the load to be lifted. *Feet First and Face It!* Squat down to the floor to lift the object onto the nearby chair.
   2. Now stand up and lift the object from the chair by straightening the hips and knees simultaneously (hip bending).
   3. Place the object on a shelf or a counter. (*Never lift above your head.*)
   4. To place an object on a shelf above your head, use a footstool or a stepladder.
D. *Lifting objects at your side with handles* (e.g., suitcase, briefcase)
   1. If possible, position yourself with your stronger side next to the object.
   2. Place your stronger side's foot ahead of your other foot.

3. Maintain a mild pelvic tilt as you bend your knees to grab the handle. Avoid twisting as you reach for the object.

4. Keep your lifting arm close to your body and your shoulders level as you straighten your knees to lift the object.

#8 COUGHING OR SNEEZING

If you feel a cough or sneeze coming on and you are in bed, bend your knees, do a mild pelvic tilt, squeeze your abdomen, and do it. If you are standing, semi-squat with your back flat against the wall, do a pelvic tilt, lock your fingers across your abdomen and squeeze, and do it. If there is no wall, do a semi-squat, a pelvic tilt, squeeze your abdomen, and do it. If you are sitting, do a pelvic tilt, flatten your back, squeeze your abdomen—*gesundheit!*

BACK PROTECTION WHILE TRAVELING

BACK FIRST, BACK FLAT, BACK STRAIGHT, BACK LAST

BACK FIRST
WHEN PACKING:

1. Allow ample time for packing at each step.

2. Keep your luggage at table height to avoid unnecessary bending. Bureaus, card tables, and dining room tables are useful for this.

3. If it is necessary to use a bed for packing, place your luggage on the bed and kneel on the floor to pack.

4. Avoid twisting, stooping, or overreaching, e.g., when unpacking, when using overhead storage areas on planes or trains, when placing carry-on luggage under seats, and when hanging garment bags in closets. Remember: *Feet First and Face It!*

BACK FLAT
WHEN LIFTING IS REQUIRED—REMEMBER:
1. to bend knees

2. to maintain a mild pelvic tilt (Back Flat)

BACK STRAIGHT
NO BENDING AT THE WAIST OR TWISTING

BACK LAST
WHEN YOU'RE CARRYING HEAVY OBJECTS:

1. Distribute the weight evenly by lifting and carrying the load with two hands.

2. Carry objects close to your body.

3. To minimize carrying, use a portable luggage "caddy" or luggage with wheels; rent a luggage cart, or hire a porter.

4. Use a backpack or shoulder straps to balance your loads.

5. Use two small suitcases rather than one large one to better distribute the weight.

6. Ask for assistance if possible.

SUPPORT YOUR BACK

1. If you are feeling slight pain or are concerned that you might stir up an old back injury, wear your corset or brace.

2. When you are getting a boarding pass or making reservations on airlines, ask for bulkhead or exit-aisle seats for more leg room. Bulkhead seats are usually reserved for families with children or for handicapped persons.

3. When making hotel reservations, ask for a firm mattress or a bedboard (*rentals may be possible from medical supply stores*). If all else fails, have someone put the mattress on the floor. If you are a FREQUENT traveler, you may want to invest in an air mattress (*and a foot pump to inflate it*).

4. Use a portable seat support, small firm pillow, blanket, towel roll, or inflatable pillow to support your low back when traveling by air, bus, car, taxi, or train.

5. Support your feet on the plane or bus by placing your feet on carry-on luggage, a purse, a briefcase, or a pillow.

6. Use carry-on luggage for a foot support when waiting in line.

7. Carry a guitar stool or Styrofoam block to support your feet when necessary.

8. Make sure your walking shoes are low-heeled, supportive, and preferably rubber-soled.

CHANGE POSITIONS OFTEN

1. When driving, stop your car often to get out and stretch your legs; WALK. When sitting, if possible, stretch by pulling one knee at a time to your chest (*see Exercise #2, pg. 227*).

2. In an airplane, get up and walk at least every hour if possible. Do mild pelvic tilts while sitting and standing; or do back bends (*see Exercise #6, pg. 234*).

PACE YOURSELF—TRY NOT TO RUSH!

1. Try to stop the activity that you are doing before your body becomes uncomfortable, tired, or painful. Pay attention to your body's message. Find a relaxing position.

2. Plan "down" time for resting time as part of your schedule. If you have been doing a lot of sitting, plan "up" or walking time.

WHAT TO DO FOR PAIN

1. Wear your corset or lumbosacral support.

2. Lie down on your back with support under your knees (*pillows, blankets, or a suitcase*), or lie on your side with a pillow between your knees.

3. Make an ice pack by putting ice in a wet towel or in a shower cap and apply to the painful area. Use ice cubes for an ice massage. Anticipate the need for a traveling cold pack (*constant ice pack or Colpac, resealable plastic bags, etc.*)

4. Take prescribed medication for pain; otherwise, take aspirin or Tylenol as directed.

5. Do these exercises:
   a. Basic Pelvic Tilt, Exercise #1 (*see pg. 225*)
   b. Single Knee to Chest, Exercise #2 (*see pg. 227*)
   c. Double Knee to Chest, Exercise #9 (*see pg. 237*)
   d. Knee Back (Lying), Exercise #7, and Knee Back (Sitting), Exercise #8 (*see pp. 235, 236*)
   e. Back Bends Standing, Exercise #6 (*see pg. 234*), if prescribed

REMEMBER: BACK FIRST—BACK FLAT—BACK STRAIGHT—BACK LAST

18.

TAKE

A BACK SEAT

BACK FIRST—BACK FLAT—BACK STRAIGHT— BACK LAST

BACK FIRST

For seating and chair selection, take a Back Seat. If you are Moderate Pain, Level 3 or Mild Pain, Level 2 (*see Table 1, "Pain Levels at a Glance," pg. 43*), choose a seat which will support your back *and* your bottom and one that you can get into and out of with relative ease. The seat should not be too high or too low, and if in doubt, choose one on the high side because it is easier to get into and out of a higher chair. For support, use a small firm pillow, a padded purse, a rolled sweater, a folded towel or table-cloth (in a restaurant), a folded newspaper or magazine, or one of several commercially available back supports. This will support the small of your back and keep it flat or slightly curved (the normal lumbar curve-in) so that you *never* have a slouching, bowed-out, or rounded back. If the seat is not firm, use a maga-zine, a disassembled cardboard box, a briefcase, a flat tray, or a commercial seat support to firm the sagging seat. Use a footstool, telephone book, suitcase, or briefcase for foot support. Avoid bench seats or seats with a partial back support that does not hit you in the small of your back. Take folding commercial back supports to the ball game, circus, and park.

If you have no choice and you must sit on a bench, then distribute your weight equally over the triangle at the bottom of your pelvis (*see Fig. 12*). This triangle consists of the angles between the bony bumps on which you sit (*ischial tuberosities*) and the bony juncture (the *symphysis pubis*) in the front of your pelvis just above your genitals (the apex of the triangle). When you are seated with your feet firmly planted on the ground or placed on a book, briefcase, or purse, etc., with your knees and hips at bent approximately 90-degree angles, your pelvis balanced in this position will help to keep you and your back straight above it. Practice this one. Try it—you'll like it!

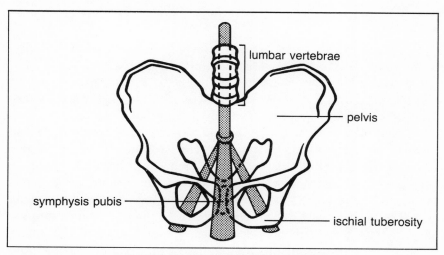

FIGURE 12 THE SEATED TRIPOD

BACK FLAT

As soon as you are aware of the slightest back discomfort, or every 20 minutes if you are in doubt, get up out of your chair. Walk around if possible. Do three to five pelvic tilts (*see Exercise #1, pg. 225.* Stand for a few minutes with one foot on a curb or with the sole of your foot or shoe placed against the wall behind you. If you can, do a few wall slides (*see Exercise #10, pg. 239*) in that position to loosen up your back muscles, and then resume sitting. If possible, improve upon your seating arrangements. Try to sit with your hips and knees slightly bent so that your knees are higher than your hips in order to keep your back flat against the back rest of your chair.

If there is no Back Seat and if you are able to squat or sit on the floor with your back against the wall, support the small of your back with a pillow, folded sweater, etc., and bend and grasp one or both knees. If you sit with your legs outstretched, your hamstring muscles (the long muscles on the backs of your thighs that stretch from the pelvis to just below the knee joint), unless they are quite loose, will pull your pelvis backwards out of the Back Flat into the Back *Strain* posture. Alternate your leg positions for comfort. Be sure you know how and *are able* to get off the floor without back strain (*see Back Protection Principle #6, pg. 157*).

BACK STRAIGHT

A comfortable chair, which allows you to sit semi-reclining with your back supported in comfort in early Moderate Pain, Level 3, is a blessing. But when you have to get *Back to Work* (*see Chapter 24*), you'll need a chair that works for your back. There are not too many things you can do sitting back, so you'll need a chair that will work with you and keep your back straight. If you have to turn and twist to function, choose a swivel chair. If you have to bend over a desk and then lean back to think, choose a tilting swivel chair. If you have to lean over your desk, work bench, or typewriter, be sure that your back support is easily adjustable, or better, designed to move to maintain back support as you lean forward or backwards. Art and drafting suppliers often have a selection, or catalogues, of adjustable seating, and they should be contacted along with office and furniture suppliers when you make your selection of a Back Seat.

BACK LAST

Choose your seat carefully. Use your arms and your legs to get in and out of it without straining your back. Always sit down under control and never flop into a chair. Adjust the height of your table, desk, or work bench so that you can get your legs underneath easily and work comfortably when sitting.

Make your back last—exercise while seated in your chair (*see* "*Exercises When Seated*," *in Chapter 27, pg 267*).

WHAT TO LOOK FOR WHEN YOU'RE GOING TO BUY A "BACK SEAT"

There is no perfect chair for everyone, nor for anyone at all times. A chair is a relatively luxurious modern device developed to provide support during work or for rest. Squatting and kneeling are still used in preference to chairs in many cultures. Squatting or kneeling encourages keeping a straight back while sitting in chairs rounds the lower back. This may explain the reported reduced incidence of disk disease in these more primitive societies.[4]

If a chair is to perform its function—or help us perform ours—it will need to be designed according to its task. A reclining chair should recline, but an executive chair should not "execute" or "kill" your back. In fact, most chairs were never designed; they just evolved from the awe inspiring thrones for royalty down to more practical plebeian items, and those that have been "designed" were created for eye appeal rather than for back support. It is only relatively recently that engineers and designers have used their skills to create seating options that can be adjusted to the individual and the function or task that she/he must perform. The draftsman's chair, the astronauts' seat, the Volvo car seat, and the modern wheelchair are some examples of good Back Seats.

THE BASIC BACK SEAT

For patients with low back pain and poor seating tolerance, the seat must be as close to ideal as possible (*see Fig. 13*). It should allow for most of the upper body weight to be supported on the back-rest of the seat. The angle of the back-rest to the seat bottom, or pan, should be about 15 degrees, gently sloping an additional 5 degrees forward at the shoulder blades in a high-backed chair. The back-rest should not push your lumbar spine too far forward into a swayback. This tends to crowd the space

[4]Fahrni, W.H., Trueman, G.E. Comparative radiological study of the spines of a primitive population with North Americans and North Europeans. Journal of Bone and Joint Surgery, 47B:552-555, 1965.

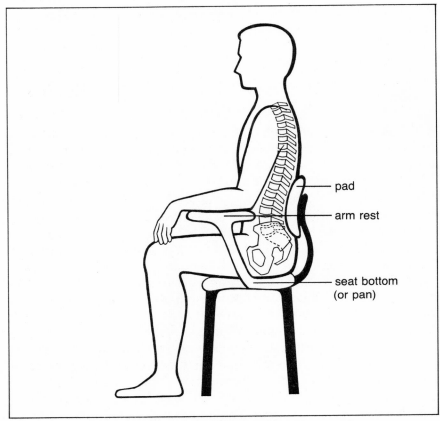

FIGURE 13 A GOOD SEAT FOR BAD BACKS

where the nerves exit between the vertebrae, and it also squeezes the facet joints together (except in those cases where the extension swayback posture has been specifically prescribed for treatment). It should also not allow you to slump or slouch in a rounded back posture because this encourages backward bulging of the disks and puts pressure on painful structures and nerves.

The area requiring maximum support is the small of your back. In typical secretarial chairs, there should be a firm pad, measuring about 6 inches or 16 centimeters in height, and 8 inches or 24 centimeters in width, which can be adjusted to fit into the small of the back. This back support, as a separate pad or built into the seat, should be firm, but not so hard or springy that it pushes out against you. Space below the firm area of back support should be sufficient to allow for your buttocks to bulge out slightly beneath the back pad or should be designed into the upholstery padding so that the buttocks are not pushed away from the back rest. The back rest should be relatively flat and not contoured or hollowed to cause rounding of the shoulders. Sagging canvas lounge chairs and deck chairs are definitely not for you if you are Moderate Pain, Level 3 to Mild Pain, Level 2.

The *chair should have arms* to allow you to use your hands when getting up and down. The arms should extend forward, preferably to the edge of the seat, so that they can be easily grasped to assist you in sitting and in pushing off when standing, especially for Moderate Pain, Level 3. The arms, preferably padded, should not be so high that your shoulders are forced upward, nor too low for the elbows to rest in comfort.

The seat bottom, or pan, should make an angle of about 15 degrees, sloping forward and upward from the back rest. It should be flat, or better, slightly scooped on each side to accommodate the buttocks. It should be wide enough to keep your thighs from rolling in and firm enough to prevent them from rolling out. By and large, if you have a "bucket" seat, you will want to bail out.

The front edge of the seat should be beveled or sloped slightly downward and padded so that the nerves and blood vessels behind the knees are not compressed between the seat edge and the bones of your legs. The seat should be firm, yet yielding sufficiently to cushion each buttock. A seat that has a firm edge but sags in the middle will cause your legs to jackknife, creating a strain on your back while seated, and will make it extremely difficult to get back up once seated. The seat should be deep enough to support your buttocks and upper thighs but should leave about 4 inches of protective clearance between the edge of the seat and the backs of your knees, unless it is a reclining chair. A low, deep "slouch couch" with wide seats is a guaranteed "ouch-couch" for your back, unless you're at Minimal Pain, Level 1.

The upholstery (fabric) should be made of a textured material or a leather that does not stick yet prevents slipping and sliding. The more you slide out of a position of comfort, the more you have to strain to get back into a good seating posture.

There should be ample room for you to place your feet and legs beneath the seat so you can have proper leg support when getting up and down.

If these features are found in the chair you already have—

great. If not, look for a chair that can be adjusted so that you can get as close to an ideal fit as possible. Remember, you can prop your chair up on blocks or purchase special blocks from medical suppliers to raise a too-low but otherwise comfortable chair to the proper height.

Don't forget to look at your old rocking chair. If it's sturdy, it can, with proper cushioning, be made into an excellent place to sit. The gentle rocking can be soothing to you, your children, your grandchildren, and above all, your back.

Now, when you are ready for more than just sitting and knitting, it is time to sit back down and think again about what your Back Seat has to do. We've swiveled and tilted in executive chairs and done the same thing with a lower profile in secretarial chairs. Remember that you want a back support pad to be right across the small of your back, just like a friendly, firm supporting hand at the back of your waist. You want that support there as much of the time as possible—when leaning back, of course, when sitting straight up, to be sure, and even when leaning forward— some chairs are specially designed with that feature in mind.

IF THE CHAIR IS ADJUSTABLE—ADJUST IT

Baby Bear just couldn't sit comfortably in Papa Bear's chair, and vice versa.

If your work requires leaning forward (looking into a CRT or microscope, or working on an assembly line), you will want a chair with a seat pan that tilts forward slightly, with a relatively shallow seat and a more beveled front.

If you work at a bench, standing and bending forward, you might do better with a tall stool that has a footrest, or a specially designed "perch" chair with a narrow seat that permits a sort of sit-stand posture with less back strain. However you adapt to your work environment, your height, weight, arm length and leg length, the seat, and your work bench or table all must be integrated so that you can work comfortably and efficiently. No chair will work for your back if there is insufficient room for your knees and legs under the desk, table, or workbench. If the chair is right and the desk is not, you may have to lower the chair arms, raise the desk, or remove a center desk drawer so that you can sit comfortably and stay *back* at work.

BACK SEAT DRIVING—CAR SEATS FOR YOUR BACK

If you are in Severe Pain, Level 4, you are a passenger. If you have a choice, pick a car with good seating. If you are in Pain Levels 3 (Moderate) through 1 (Minimal) and are in the market for a new car, pick one with an "up front Back Seat." Volvo was the first to actually design a car seat for back support and back protection. More and more automobile manufacturers are paying attention to seating, and your choice of cars with well designed seats is broadening each year (let's hope *your* seat is not!). Avoid bucket seats and particularly those seats with raised edges and projecting sides. Getting in and out of such seats, particularly in a low-slung, sporty car, can get your back out of the driving scene. Avoid sleek, slippery upholstered surfaces because you will strain your back trying to stay put. Low seats that force your feet straight out in front of you are stressful to your back while you are sitting and worse when getting in and getting out. If your car looks sharp but sitting in it stabs you in the back, borrow or rent another car until your back is better.

If you are satisfied with your car but need to upgrade the seats, you should consider installing custom seats. Custom seating requires careful selection. Most manufacturers of custom car seats can provide you with well designed and supportive seating, but showrooms and automotive accessory dealers tend to emphasize seats designed for racing or for eye appeal. Don't get a racy seat unless you are a racer. Be sure your seat is wide enough and has no (or minimal) edge lips and projections. Look for an adjustable lumbar support or a customized comfortable lumbar support. All adjustment knobs and levers designed to move the seat forward and backward, raise or lower it, or increase or decrease the angle of incline should be accessible and easily manipulated.

If you are at Moderate Pain, Level 3 or Mild Pain, Level 2, you should take a Back Seat. Sit close, sit straight, bend your knees and not your back.

Seat cushion springs must be firm for support, otherwise you might sink in and jackknife your thighs, never to ride again. Shock absorbers and tire pressure should be optimal. If you have a yen for the open road, be sure it is smoothly paved or the *road back* will be a long, hard one.

In our experience, the best all around seat support to place in your car in order to make marginal or poor seating into good seating is the Sacro-Ease Car Seat. If you purchase this seat support, be sure that it is bent just right to support the small of your back when you are actually in your car. If you need to improvise to make a poor seat into a tolerable one, use a disassembled cardboard box, several magazines, a briefcase, or a flat tray underneath you; use a firm pillow, a folded newspaper, or a rolled towel behind the small of your back for support.

If you're at Severe Pain, Level 4 or Moderate Pain, Level 3, and you're ready for your first outing or drive, be sure the trip you plan will not require you to sit for more than half of the time that you have been able to sit comfortably at home. In other words, if you can sit only for 30 minutes in a good chair at home, don't plan a drive longer than 15 minutes.

If you're a passenger and you're at Moderate Pain, Level 3, try the exercise for sitting in the car about every 10 minutes (*see pg. 164*). If you are the driver, do the exercises at each stop, or stop every 20 minutes and do them. At first it is best to stop the car about every 20 minutes, get out, walk around, and do some pelvic tilts (*see pg. 225*) and wall slides (*see pg. 253*). You may gather a few interested gawkers, but it's worth it. At Mild Pain, Level 2, as your back condition improves and your sitting tolerance grows, you can extend the time between stops. It's never a good idea to drive for more than two hours at a stretch, even if you are doing the sitting exercises en route.

GETTING BACK IN AND OUT AND BACK ON THE ROAD

The whole trip can be off if getting in the car gets you in the *back*. So let's *back* into this trip carefully.

BACK FIRST

If you're at Moderate Pain, Level 3, sit in the front seat on your first outing, unless you plan to lie down in back.

STEP I   Be sure the car seat you have chosen is as close to ideal as possible.

STEP II   Be sure that the seat is pushed back as far as it can be to provide ample room for getting into the car.

STEP III   Open the car door (if you are still in a lot of pain, have someone else open it). Be sure the car is parked so that there is enough room to get in and out. Use any convenient part of the door, roof, or frame, or a cane as a hand support. Turn around and place the backs of your legs against the car.

BACK FLAT

Do a pelvic tilt and lower yourself slowly to the seat using your arms and legs. Raise your feet one at a time onto the edge of the car. You may find it easier to lift one or both legs with your hand. Use one hand over the car's rain gutter and one on the seat to support yourself. Keeping your back as straight as possible, move your legs slowly in a 90-degree arc until you are sitting and facing straight ahead. If you have to be the driver, move the seat forward as close to the steering wheel as is comfortable. Fasten your seatbelt, but do it carefully, without twisting.

SPECIAL REMINDERS

If you're at Moderate Pain, Level 3 to Mild Pain, Level 2 and you do a lot of stop-and-go driving, try to use a car with an automatic transmission and power brakes. If you've got packages to load and unload, keep them small and light and place them close to the door. If they are bulky, use the trunk—it's difficult, but the Back Seat in a two-door car is worse for reaching in and out. (*Review Back Protection Principle #7, pg. 159.*)

IF YOU HAVE TO LOAD AND UNLOAD THE TRUNK:

■ *Back First.* If you're at Moderate Pain, Level 3 to Mild Pain, Level 2, place a small box or crate bottom-up on the floor of your trunk if needed to raise the bottom so that you will not have to reach so far in. If you have a station wagon, arrange the packages so that they stay close to the hatch.

■ *Back Flat.* Stand as close as possible to the rear bumper with your feet under the bumper, keeping your knees slightly bent and holding a pelvic tilt.

■ *Back Straight.* Place one foot under the bumper and bend from your hips, keeping your back straight (*see Back Protection Principle #4, pg. 155*). Hold any packages as close to your chest as possible. If you are tall (or the car is small), you can try putting one foot on the bumper or actually into the trunk.

■ *Back Last.* Use your arms and legs to lift the parcel. Use the back ledge of the trunk as a temporary shelf and lift the load in stages—first to the edge of the trunk, then into the trunk, and vice versa when removing objects. Store objects as close to the rear of the trunk as possible.

19.

BACK IN BED

What should you know before purchasing the bed and mattress in which you will spend one third of the *rest* of your life?

Bedrest is essential to back pain management. The bed you rest in and the way you get in and out of it may make or break the success of this essential component of back pain therapy.

THE MATTRESS

You may be spending a lot of time in bed for a while, so spend it wisely and well.

The mattress should be firm but should compress and indent sufficiently in areas where the body has bulges (the buttocks) to allow the body to assume essentially the same configuration when lying on your back as when standing. When side-lying, the mattress should allow for indentation at the shoulder, hip, and knees sufficient to keep the body in a straight line. The mattress must not be lumpy or sag if postural strain is to be prevented.

HARDNESS

If the mattress is too firm, the body protrusions at the buttocks and shoulders are not accommodated and the back is forced to arch between them, causing strain. A hard mattress also presses against bony prominences, which may become tender as a result.

SOFTNESS

If the mattress gives way, it is difficult to turn over and get in and out of bed. The edge of the mattress of the right firmness should sink approximately two inches when sat upon.

FOAM PADDING

Most mattresses have a thin upper layer of padding or foam rubber. Mattresses made entirely of high density polyurethane foam rubber that is too dense may push up against the body protrusions, creating a strain. Therefore, medium density polyurethane foam should be selected. As a rule of thumb, each mattress manufacturer has its own guidelines for degree of firmness, which can vary from year to year. A medium-firm mattress is usually about right, depending on your weight and/or that of your partner. Try lying on a mattress for at least 20 minutes before deciding if it is really comfortable.

BED HEIGHT

With the mattress and box springs on a conventional bed, the mattress top should be about two feet from the ground for ease in getting in and out, and for bed-making as well. This may vary by several inches up or down, depending on your height.

BED FRAME

This should be made of heavy duty metal, with deep supporting edges and at least one central support bar to prevent the mattress from sagging. A queen size bed should have at least six legs with 2½ inch rug guard casters for ease in moving. For acute care of a severe level of pain, a hospital bed with power adjustable leg and head elevators as well as an adjustable overall bed height is ideal for ease in positioning and ease in getting in and out. Make sure that you get a reasonably new, firm (not extra-firm) mattress. The use of short siderails attached to the bed, or of an overhead trapeze bar, can also facilitate position changes in bed. Adjustable electric beds, which are divided into two parts for individual adjustment, can be obtained in king size and queen size versions. These beds usually do not have a high-low height adjustment feature. Hospital beds and adjustable electric beds may be rented or purchased at a medical or surgical supply store (if you're renting, insist that your mattress is in top condition).

WATERBEDS

If you don't get seasick (some people actually get seasick on a waterbed), these mattresses can be very comfortable. A heated waterbed is a cozy one. Changing positions in a waterbed is more difficult than on a conventional mattress, and getting in and out can be extremely tricky. I know of no way to predict who will be comfortable and who will be miserable on a waterbed. One group most apt to be comfortable is those who like to sleep on their backs. Waterbeds are becoming increasingly more sophisticated and many contain baffles to channel the water. The more they are baffled, the less they function as a flotation device. If you have been sold on a waterbed, don't buy it until you try one for the night, perhaps at a motel. It may not exactly be a vacation, but it may save your back for the rest of your life.

THE FLOOR, THE "I'D RATHER BE DEAD THAN IN BED" MATTRESS

The floor, to say the least, is unyielding. A mattress on the floor may be better than a sagging mattress on a bed. It will never be as good as a good mattress on a bed, unless you are sleeping on a Japanese type futon mattress. Remember, getting on and off the floor can be painful, so you'd better know how to execute these maneuvers without straining your back before trying to rest on the floor (*see Back Protection Principle #6, pg. 157*).

HOW TO UNSAG THE MATTRESS

BED BOARDS

Bed boards inserted between the box spring and mattress can help relieve mattress sag. They should be at least ½" thick if you weigh less than 125 pounds, ¾" thick if you weigh more than 125 pounds, and 1" thick if you weigh more than 225 pounds. They should be long enough and wide enough to support you from the shoulders to the knees (at least 3' by 4'). If you are traveling, ask for one in your hotel. If they don't have a bed board and the mattress is not satisfactory, ask them to place it on the floor. The purpose of the bed board, to keep your mattress from sagging, can often be accomplished almost as well by sliding (get someone to help you) a 1 x 1½" board or dowel or broom handle under the mattress (above the box springs) at the level of your hips, and another at the level of your shoulders. A third board or dowel under the knees may be necessary to prevent further sagging.

RECLINING IN BED

A hospital bed or adjustable bed is ideal for this, but you can substitute a foam wedge bolster or obtain a "slant" board. Or, you can improvise one with a card table and place a "cascade" of pillows between you and the headboard or wall for support in the reclining position.

PILLOWS

Use small down pillows or similar polyester-fiber pillows. Avoid large foam rubber pillows except for placement between your legs for support in the side-lying position and under your knees for comfort when you are lying on your back. When you put them under your head, they tend to push the head into a strained position, and since the neck connects the head to the back, this may head you back into back pain.

SHOULD I BUY A NEW MATTRESS?

The average mattress should be turned monthly for the first six months and then every three months if it is going to live its life expectancy. If it has had good care, it may last ten to twenty years. If yours has not, and it is over five years old, and if you are waking up in the morning stiff and achy, you'd better think about a new mattress.

MATTRESS FEATURES

The mattress should be about six inches thick to keep it from bottoming out. It should be light, and it should have two handles sturdily sewn into each side for ease in turning. If it is a foam mattress, it may be constructed with different densities of polyurethane to maintain level support under body parts to different weights such as the head, shoulders, buttocks, and feet. The ticking (the outer cover) should be sewn to the foam or springs to prevent it from slipping. The mattress should have a low frequency of oscillation (less bounce to the ounce); the edges should be firm for ease in getting in and out. The springs should be noiseless, or as close to that as possible. There should be no odor to the mattress, and it should be well insulated to prevent heat accumulation or chilling. Polyurethane mattresses should be made of solid sheets rather than from shredded polyurethane, which has poor durability.

MATTRESS COILS AND SPRINGS

The firmness of a conventional mattress is a function of the number of springs and the thickness of the wire. An "orthopedic" mattress may have from 500 to 700 coils, with springs ranging in gauge from 12½ (heavy-durable) to 15½ gauge. The box (supports about 40% of the body weight) should match the springs. The box has roughly a fourth the number of springs and they are of a heavy 9 gauge. The typical mattress has knotted coil ends. The cloth "pocketed" coil is somewhat subject to tearing and displacement.

Mattresses are sold by their manufacturer's name ("ortho" this and "posture" that) with the implication that they are uniquely posture supporting or orthopedically ideal. The mattress cover is its eye appeal, but the typical floral design is not visible when the bed is made. So try the mattress; ask to see its inner construction. Know at least the approximate number of coils that you are buying. Be sure (do a 20-minute test) that you are comfortable and can get in and out of it, and if the price is right—buy it!

20.

SAFELY

BACK HOME:

GETTING THROUGH

THE DAY

There's no place like home. True, but if you have a back problem, you may have to make some adjustments. Familiar surroundings are taken for granted. Inconveniences such as stuck windows, overstuffed chairs, or dark stairwells become a part of life and the problems go unnoticed. You may be aggravating your back in a dozen ways every day without realizing it. We call this "wasting pain." If a strained back can tolerate five minor strains before going into spasm, don't use up that precious reserve by straining your back unnecessarily.

DON'T WASTE PAIN!

Lubricate all doors, drawers, and windows. If they're stuck, try to get someone else to open them. If you can't get help, push rather than pull whenever possible. Always use basic back-protection reaching and lifting techniques (*see Chapter 17*).

Leave nothing to slip on or trip over on the floor or stairs. Have no highly polished floors or throw rugs. Always have secure footing for whatever your task. Light your way at night. You don't need to trip—it could be the start of a trip to the hospital.

Organize closets and shelves to avoid reaching up, reaching out, or squatting down. Have stools and ladders available. A stool a fool forgets, and the latter a ladder as well.

Stairs beware. Organize your day to minimize trips up and down. If you're hurting, use the railing for support. Descend stairs "down with the bad" leg (the leg on the most painful side) first, and ascend "up with the good" leg. Touch the stair toe-first on the step down. Try to get as much of your foot as possible on the stair, and get both feet on one step before proceeding up or down to the next.

Wheels. Use wheels (carts, wagons, or wheelbarrows) to carry loads. Travel light and make several trips rather than overload and strain your back.

THE BED AND BEDROOM

SEVERE PAIN, LEVEL 4

The bed should be located downstairs (*stairs beware*). The bed height, with the mattress, should be about three inches above your knees for easy access (*see Chapter 19*). Use a short siderail, an overhead trapeze, a portable adjustable vertical pole, or a bedside table. The best bed is an electric-powered high-low adjustable hospital bed with a good mattress. Use power to flatten your mattress, then support your back by raising the head of the bed until you reach a sitting position. Using your hands for support, swing your legs over the side of the bed and stand (*see Back Protection Principle #2, pg. 151*). Don your corset if you have one (*see Chapter 15, pg. 132*), preferably in bed.

Leave nothing on the floor to slip on or trip over.

Bed-making: Someone else will have to do it.

Exercise in bed (*see pg. 184*).

SEVERE PAIN, LEVEL 4 TO MODERATE PAIN, LEVEL 3

A downstairs bed location is still preferred (*see Back Protection Principle #2, pg. 151; see Chapter 19*). An electric blanket makes it easier to stay warm in bed without twisting to pull heavy blankets and quilts. Organize closets and shelves for easy access to clothes. Keep essentials between elbow and shoulder height.

■ *Exercise in Bed.* Exercise in bed before arising—start out easy. Do three gentle pelvic tilts (*see pg. 225*) and three alternating knee-chest exercises (*see pg. 227*); then do three double knee-chests (*see pg. 237*); and finally, three beginning pelvic rotations (*see pg. 244*) just to make sure that everything is working before getting up.

MODERATE PAIN, LEVEL 3 TO MINIMAL PAIN, LEVEL 1

Exercise on the floor. If the carpet is padded and the room is not drafty, the floor is the best place to do your exercises, unless you have difficulty getting up and down (*see Back Protection Principle #6, pg. 157*). A small exercise mat can be placed on a rug or hardwood floor for additional padding and then folded and put away if need be. An electric blanket is a good floor warmer.

■ *Corset.* Don in bed if getting up is painful (*see "Corsets," pg. 132*).

■ *Bed-making.* If you must do it, do it on your knees and keep your back straight. If you have a large bed, you may have to lean on one hand or even lie across the bed to reach across it to straighten the spread or adjust pillows.

THE CLOTHES ON YOUR BACK

SEVERE PAIN, LEVEL 4

■ *Dressing*—Stay in your bedclothes unless you must go out to see the doctor.

Clothes—Lay them out in an accessible place or on a coat rack or valet. Choose loose-fitting and easily adjustable clothes; jogging suits are perfect. Twisting for hard to reach zippers or buttons and pulling tight clothes on from below or above may put your back out. Dress appropriately for the weather. Neither chilling nor sweltering will help.

Closets—All clothes should be hung at elbow to shoulder

height and unnecessary clothing packed away so that what you need can be easily removed and replaced.

Loose-fitting slacks—For women, loose slacks make squatting easier in social situations—you can keep your legs apart.

Belts—Belts should be placed on pants before pants are put on. Twisting to get the belt through the loops is asking your back for trouble.

Bras—Front-closing bras are best. Put shoulders through straps, place one foot on a stool, keep your back straight, and lean forward from the hips, letting your breasts fill the cups. To fasten, do a pelvic tilt and stand up. Bras that attach from behind should be attached in front first, then twisted around before slipping your arms through the straps.

Underpants and panty hose—(Don't use panty hose until your back problem is no worse than Moderate Pain, Level 3.) These are best put on *in bed lying on your back* with one knee bent. If you have more pain on one side, put the "good" leg in first so it can help stabilize you. You don't want to strain your back while trying to get the painful leg through the hole. Pull the underpants or pants partway up before placing the second leg through its hole. Next best, don your underpants and hose standing and leaning with your back against a wall. A chair or high stool for leg support helps. Reacher-sticks, a stretched-out wire hanger as a hook, and even canes can help you grab or pick up objects on the floor and are very handy in dressing maneuvers. Remember the Four Back Words (*see pg. 63*) and remember: "good leg first."

Pants—The same rules apply as for underpants. Tight elastic waistbands are not worth the struggle.

Stockings—Put stockings on in bed like underpants, or sitting or standing with your foot on a stool. Specially designed stocking donners that extend your reach can be purchased (try a medical or surgical equipment supply house, or a pharmacy) to make this task less formidable in the sitting or standing position.

Shoes—Use slip-on slippers indoors. Loafers or slip-on shoes are easiest to get on and off for outdoor wear. Use a long-handled shoehorn and place your foot on a stool, chair seat, or counter so you won't have to bend your back to get into your shoes. Elastic shoelaces that don't require tying can make an ordinary shoe function like a loafer. You will still need to use a long-handled shoehorn. Boots are out. They are too hard to get on and off.

Heels—The maximum height is 1″, and they should be of moderate-firm rubber for cushioning. Too soft a heel or sole can make your foot wiggle and your back writhe.

Soles—A moderately firm rubber sole cushions the shock of each step.

MODERATE PAIN, LEVEL 3 TO MILD PAIN, LEVEL 2

■ *Shoes*. High heels greater that 1¼″ are best avoided. They cause swayback and make balance difficult. Any shoe that pinches or otherwise causes foot discomfort should be avoided because you will walk differently to avoid the foot pain, and the result can be back strain. A supportive shoe for walking, with 4 to 5 laces and a firm counter (the part of the shoe that supports the side and back of your heel), is what you are looking for.

BATHROOM

SEVERE PAIN, LEVEL 4

■ *Toilet*. Get a raised toilet seat for temporary use, available at your surgical supply house.

Handrails—Use attachable toilet-seat handrails, or counters and sinks, for support. Ease onto the seat, don't plop down.

Position—Sit with your back straight, lean forward from your hips (*see Back Protection Principle #3, pg. 152*). Place one or both feet flat on a small stool in front of you. For some people, squatting with both feet on the toilet seat works best. Grasp the front of your knees or push down on them for additional support. Be sure and have someone help you if you want to try this one.

Paper—Toilet paper should be retrievable without twisting. If not, take what you need before you are seated, or just put the toilet paper roll in your lap.

Flush—If the flush-handle is not accessible when you're sitting, stand up, keeping your back straight, and face the handle. Bend your hips and knees; support yourself with one hand, and reach with the other (step forward with the leg on the "reaching" side) to flush. Or, use a stretched-out clothes hanger, a cane, or a string (pull the chain) to minimize the stretch. In some toilets, it is easier to stand with your weight on the good leg and use the opposite foot to flush.

■ *Sink*. Remember the Four Back Words. Use the highest available counter; or place a drawer (upside down), a box, or a small suitcase on the counter to increase the surface height of the one you have. Place your toilet articles on the elevated surface. This will lessen your need to bend over.

■ *Toothbrush and Cup*. Fill your cup or glass full to avoid refilling and more bending. Use a long flexible straw to minimize bending and a plastic bib in case you're messy.

■ *Shower*. Lubricate your shower door: You don't want to jerk it open. Use a shower head with a hose attached for easier access.

Water temperature—Adjust the water temperature before entering the shower. If you don't, you and your back might both go out in hurry. Be sure that your shower pan has a non-skid surface. Also, warm the bathroom before disrobing.

Shower shelves—Soap, shampoo, and sponges should be placed on the shelves in the shower at elbow to shoulder height. Keep duplicates of essentials in case something drops, and if it drops, leave it. A soap-on-a-rope that can be hung around your neck and will reach around to your back is handy, and a long-handled scrub brush is a great back saver.

Shower stools—Stools should be non-skid, water resistant, and tall enough for easy sitting. A lower step for foot placement is an additional back pain reliever.

Shower wall—Spray the wall to take away the chill (you should have an easily adjusted shower head), and then flatten your back and assume a partial knee-bend position with your feet about 12 inches apart. Support your back against the wall, facing the shower.

Shampoo—Use the shower wall for back support, and rinse facing the shower head. A shower head on a hose attachment can help you rinse without straining. In either case, face the shower head, do a mild pelvic tilt, bend your hips and knees, and remember the Four Back Words.

Legs and feet—Support your back against the wall. Use a shower stool, and place one foot at a time on the stool. Use a

long-handled sponge to assist in soaping. If this is still too difficult, just let the water rinse your legs and feet clean.

■ *Tub.* If you can't get out—don't go in! Be sure that there is a
non-skid mat or bottom in your tub. Use an adjacent counter or
sink for hand-support or, better yet, handrails attached to the tub
and/or "grab" bars attached to the wall.

Water temperature—Water temperature should be 102 degrees maximum. Spend no more than 5 to 10 minutes in the tub,
because prolonged sitting in a tub rounds your back, and the
warmth, while relaxing, is weakening. Moreover, getting back up
may become impossible, and you could be back down again. If no
shower is available, get a shower hose extension for the tub,
preferably for use while sitting on a stool in the tub or on a board
placed across it. If you are only going to partly submerge, be sure
the bathroom is well heated.

Getting back out—Either reverse the process of getting in,
or let most of the water out and then turn on your hands and
knees and crawl up and out.

The ring—Let someone else, or a bubble bath, clean it if
possible.

■ *Drying.* Put on a terry cloth robe to dry your body, and step on
a towel to dry your feet. Next best, use a large, absorbent towel
for your body, and dry your feet by putting them one at a time on
a towel placed on a stool, chair, toilet seat, or sink. Keep a second
towel handy in case the first one drops. Try a hair dryer instead
of a towel.

MODERATE PAIN, LEVEL 3 TO MILD PAIN, LEVEL 2

■ *Toilet.* Look over the toilet tips for Severe Pain, Level 4, and
use any that you find helpful.

■ *Sink.* Choose any of the tips for Severe Pain, Level 4 that
make it easier to avoid back strain.

■ *Grooming.* Use an adjustable mirror that can be pulled close to
your face for makeup or shaving. An electric razor can be used in
bed, and that is best. Stand with your feet on a low stool, or on a
box placed under the sink, or open a door or drawer beneath the

sink and step on the ledge to keep your back flat. Lean one hand on the counter for support whenever possible.

■ *Medicine Cabinet.* Put necessary medicines, vitamins, etc., on the most accessible shelf (between elbow and shoulder height), or better, put them out on your elevated counter top within easy reach.

■ *Shower.* Look over the tips for Severe Pain, Level 4, and use whatever makes it easier for you to spare your back. If you're going to remodel, place the shower faucet knobs at elbow height and within easy reach from the door for water temperature and force adjustment. Adjustable showerhead massage jets are a pleasant option. Wall slides can be easily done before leaving the shower (*see Chapter 28, "The Five-Minute Back Saver"*).

■ *Tub.* Too long a tub-bath can leave you weak, weary, and worry your back. Jets and Jacuzzis feel nice, but cure nothing. Just be sure you can get back out without slipping.

■ *Drying.* Use what's useful from Severe Pain, Level 4 if you need it, and remember the Four Back Words.

■ *Blow Dry Hair.* Blow dry your hair using the same techniques as for grooming, or better, use an electric hair-dryer hat.

21.

HELPFUL

HOUSEHOLD HINTS

FOR ALL

PAIN LEVELS

THE KITCHEN

Calories do count, and so does your back. Bending down and reaching into the depths of the refrigerator for a quart of low fat milk may reduce you to a state of misery. Remember the Four Back Words (*see pg. 63*). Pace yourself to avoid overwork, fatigue, or prolonged standing or sitting. Change tasks and positions frequently. Walk around. Lie down. Do five pelvic tilts (*see Exercise #1, pg. 225*) while standing, and if you can do so comfortably, do five back bend exercises to relieve low back tension and strain (*see Exercise #6, pg. 234; see Back Protection Principles #5 and #7, pp. 156, 159*).

■ *Refrigerators and Freezers.* Store heavier bulky items on top shelves, and keep essentials in easily seen and easily reached locations.

■ *Counters and Cupboards.* Store all essentials within easy reach on the counter. Slide whatever needs moving, and don't lift if you can avoid it. The ideal counter height is 2 to 3 inches below the bottom of your elbows when you are standing.

Heavy objects, pots, pans, and packages should all be placed on the counter if possible or as close to counter-level as they can be.

Light objects are stored above. Use a *stepstool or ladder* to reach them.

Medium weight objects can be stored below if necessary. Squat or kneel to lift (*see Back Protection Principles #5 and #7, pp. 156, 159*).

■ *Cooking.* Stand with one foot on a small stool or on the lower edge of an open cupboard or emptied bottom drawer beneath the sink. Place one hand or elbow on the counter and press down on it while leaning (bend the hips) over the counter (*see Back Protection Principle #4, pg. 155*). Lift pots with two hands if sliding on the counter will not work. Lift a pot, pan, or package off of the counter and close to your chest by facing the object and moving it toward you, keeping your back flat and straight with your knees and hips bent—lift with your legs (*see Back Protection Principle #7, pg. 159*). If this is awkward, slide the object toward your "good side" and lift, as above, holding the object close to your side. This will cause you to lean away from the pain, and you may get the job done without back strain. If you carry a lifted object, face the new location feet first (*see Feet First and Face It! pg. 150*).

■ *Wheels and Carts.* These should be used for all carrying. Any objects lifted, including the entire meal you've prepared, should be placed on a tall cart and wheeled to the table or wherever necessary.

■ *Devices.* Mechanical can and jar openers and grinders are essential, but if you are in severe pain, purchase pre-cooked meals and avoid the whole meal-preparation hassle, including washing dishes. Use your dishwasher if it is easy to fill and empty. If not, then just rinse your dishes. Remember the Four Back Words.

■ *Eating.* Take a Back Seat (*see Back Protection Principle #3, pg. 152*).

Good manners—Avoid reaching across the table.

Bad manners (but good body mechanics)—lean on your elbow when eating. The weight supported on your arm means less strain on the lower disks.

TELEPHONE

Place the phone in an easily accessible location at a comfortable height. Don't trip over the extension cord. Get a message recorder so you won't have to run when the phone rings. Use a speaker phone, if possible.

LAUNDRY

The Four Back Words and *Feet First and Face It!* are essential if you are to avoid dirty words when your back starts hurting in the laundry. Lifting or dragging more than you can easily handle so you won't have to make an extra trip is a "lazy man's" load when you've got back trouble that can put you back in bed! Use wheels, or slide your laundry load. Wet clothes are heavy, so empty the washing machine in stages. Bending, stooping, and lifting are very stressful, so rest between loads. Do 2 to 5 pelvic tilts or back bends if you know that you can do them comfortably (*see "Feel-Good" Easing Exercises, pg. 263*) after each load.

■ *Ironing.* Use a high ironing board. Lean against a wall with your knees bent, or stand with one foot on a stool beneath the ironing board. Better yet, send the laundry out for awhile.

UPSTAIRS, DOWNSTAIRS

Stay in one place (on one floor) as much as possible. Organize your activities so you will need to make as few trips up and down the stairs as possible. Rent an extra bed (hospital type) if need be, and turn the living room into a temporary bedroom. Use the railing, the wall, or a cane for support when going up and down the stairs. Step down with the "bad leg" (the leg on the most painful side) and up with the "good" one. Place as much of your foot as possible on each step, and place both feet on one step before going on to the next.

■ *Vacuum Cleaners.* Vacuum cleaners, mops, brooms, and long-handled dustpans are needed for both upstairs and downstairs—so have two sets if possible. When vacuuming, mopping, etc., keep your back flat and straight, and lean forward at the hips, stepping smoothly forward with the mop or vacuum cleaner much like a fencer steps forward when he lunges. If you can mop or vacuum with one hand, step forward with the same hand and leg.

TRASH

Use barrels on wheels (or on a wagon or wheelbarrow). Avoid lifting clumsy heavy trash and trash containers. A trash compressor can help you manage your trash. Bundle your trash into small manageable packages. Make several trips with small bundles rather than juggling one large or bulky bundle. The idea that you can carry or drag one large load all at once and get it over with is really the lazy man's way and the risky way for your back. Don't carry a "lazy man's load."

BABY'S ROOM

■ *Crib.* Keep the mattress as high as possible. Lower the crib rail before lifting. Slide the baby; or if the baby is old enough, have the baby come close before being lifted (*see Back Protection Principle #7, pg. 159*).

■ *Footstool.* Place a footstool under the crib and Bathinette, or place your foot in the space left by the removal of a bottom bureau drawer.

■ *Chair.* Take a Back Seat (*see Chapter 18*). Support the baby in your lap when possible.

■ *Carrying.* A backpack is best, but a front pouch or sling holding the baby as close to your body as possible will work well for a few months. Keep your back straight, and bend only from the hips and knees.

■ *Stairs Beware*. Keep the baby and baby activities on the same floor level as your own.

LIVING ROOM AND/OR DEN

If you have a reasonably firm favorite lounge chair, you might be able to make a Back Seat out of it by placing a firm pillow or rolled towel in the small of your back and putting your legs up on the seat of a breakfast or dining room chair.

■ *Relaxing*. This sounds great, but if you don't pick your spot well, your back can sink into a hole that you can't crawl out of. What looks *great*—deep, padded lounge chairs or low, slick couches—are sure to slowly *grate* your spine. Stay away from couches and you will avoid the classic "couch-ouch" that hits you in the back when you try to get *back* up. Take a Back Seat.

■ *TV Viewing*. How you watch TV can either work for you or against you. Choose a Back Seat! Line the TV up for comfortable viewing. If you wear bifocals, have the TV at a height so that you can avoid eye strain, neck strain, and back strain. Keep the TV tuned for sharp focus, and if your back pain is moderate or severe, get a remote control box.

■ *Sewing Machine*. Take a Back Seat! Secure good lighting. Raise the sewing machine on blocks if necessary so that you can work without bending your back.

■ *Furniture*. If your furniture needs rearranging, get help. If you must, push at shoulder height to roll or slide furniture. Remember the Four Back Words. Use a dolly whenever possible. If it's a two-man job, rehearse the process, so both of you know what to expect—before "it" happens to your *back*.

PAPER WORK

Take a Back Seat.

■ *Reading*. Secure good lighting. Wear glasses if you need them. Consider a desktop book stand so that you can read without bending. Be sure that there is clearance for your knees under your desk. Central desk drawers usually crowd your legs and will strain your back. A drafting table makes a good work desk. You can adjust the legs for optimal table height and then tilt the entire tabletop for easy access. Bricks, wood blocks, or special table-leg extenders can raise the entire desk or be placed under the back legs to tilt the desktop for easier reach and reading.

■ *Writing*. Take a Back Seat and adjust your lighting. If you take pen in hand, there is usually no problem. Typewriting is another story. A Back Seat, good lighting, leg room, and comfortable keyboard positioning are essential. A book stand for reference reading or transcription can make the job easier.

■ *Arithmetic*. Add up all the costs of any suggestions you've purchased in *Good News for Bad Backs*—it's worth it!

IN THE BACK YARD

■ *In and Out the Door*. Push the door (or gate) open. Stand close to the door, and walk with it as it opens, for balance.

If you must pull the door open, first stand close, then bend your knees, keeping your back straight and your elbows at your sides. Step to the door, grasp the knob, and pull without jerking.

THE GARDEN

Once you are back in the back yard, it is definitely time to cultivate good back habits. The Four Back Words are indispensable. Face every task *feet first*. Pivot by moving your feet and not by twisting your trunk. If you want to see your garden grow, divide the workload, and do what has to be done in easy stages. If you want to watch a blooming weed patch from your bedroom, hurry up and groan. Much of garden work requires bending and stooping. If you can do the standing back-extension exercise (*see Exercise #6, pg. 234*), you may find that standing upright and performing ten repetitions of this exercise every 10 to 20 minutes can keep you going and the garden growing. But pace yourself anyway. Walking around and changing your posture and activity every 10 to 20 minutes is also a good back saver. Five to ten pelvic tilts while standing also helps loosen tight back muscles.

Let's look at some typical gardening tasks, problems, and solutions. Keep in mind that any digging should be done in soil that has been moistened for softness but not allowed to become soggy and heavy with water. Be sure that all cutting and digging tools are sharp and all mechanical parts work smoothly.

■ *Weeding and Planting.* This usually requires kneeling, although long-handled weeders are available and much weeding can be done standing. To ease the kneeling position, use a low padded stool, a foam knee cushion, or knee pads. When kneeling, the shock absorbing function of the foot, ankle, and knee is not in effect, and the stress from your arms goes directly to your back and hips. Kneeling on one knee and pressing one hand on the ground gives added support. If you can't kneel comfortably, try sitting on a low stool or squatting "native" style, and use a long-handled weeder. In these positions, the hips are almost out of action so Back Straight (*see Back Protection Principle #1, pg. 148*) and Hip Bend (*see Back Protection Principle #4, pg. 155*) are even more crucial to back protection.

■ *Raking and Hoeing.* The technique for raking is similar to that for vacuuming. Keep your back straight and bend your knees and hips in a smooth easy lunging motion. If the raking job is a heavy one, get a blower to assist you. Hoe with your arms close to your body, keeping your back straight, and let the bent hips and knees take the load.

Look for lightweight, long-handled garden tools with a two-hand grasp attachment for easier handling. You may also find bent-angled handles on a variety of tools designed for a stronger grasp and less back and arm strain.

■ *Shoveling.* Use sharpened shovels in properly prepared soil. Support the shovel handle with one hand at mid-shaft to ease the lifting effort. Keep the load close to the body. Use slow, rhythmical movements, bending at the knees and hips and keeping the back straight. Turn to dump the load by pivoting with your feet to keep your trunk from twisting. *Feet First and Face It!* Don't shovel snow. Get a blower to do it.

■ *Pruning.* Use a ladder and a long-handled, sharp pruner or power trimmers. Don't lean back. If you can't clip easily, get a better tool, or better—get help. Intersperse pruning with raking and resting. It's the job you want to finish—not your back.

■ *Wheelbarrows.* Grease the axle! Use proper lifting techniques (*see Back Protection Principle #7 pg. 159*). Don't carry a "lazy man's load."

■ *Lawn Mowing.* Get a power mower with a starter switch. Don't use a jerk cord for starting; it can stop you—in the back.

BACK IN THE GARAGE AND WORKSHOP

Whether you're back in the garage, in the basement, on the roof, or under the house, the basic principles of back protection apply. The Four Back Words are foremost. Pacing, by varying your jobs, will help you avoid over-strain from any one activity or posture. Turning your whole body, by pivoting with your feet to avoid twisting your back, means that you face a project feet first to begin (*Feet First and Face It!*). When the completed project needs to be moved, you avoid twisting your back by turning your whole body feet first and facing the new place where you will deposit your load. If the task has to be done lying down under the car or under the house, change your body position by log-rolling (moving your hips, trunk, and shoulders as a unit) when turning from side to side. Remember that you can strain yourself almost as easily by twisting to pick up the mail or a leaf as you can by lifting a heavy log. Review Back Protection Principles #7 (*see pg. 159*) and #6 (*see pg. 157*).

Be sure to lubricate your garage door, or better yet, get an automatic garage door opener. Keep all tools within easy reach and in smooth working order. Get the right tools for each job. The money you spend on proper equipment, you will save on your back.

■ *Lifting and Carrying.* Make sure that you have secure footing. Avoid slick, wet, or greasy surfaces. If a load is bulky or heavy, get help. If you are going to assist in lifting and carrying, rehearse the whole process, *then clear the path.* Be sure all doors are easily opened and negotiable, and that the path is clear—also that the steps are manageable and that rest stops can be made. Lift *smoothly*. The actual lift should not be undertaken unless it can be smoothly executed and body position changes en route can be done by pivoting with your feet and not by twisting.

■ *Balance the Load.* It is better to carry two small bucket loads, one in each hand, then one heavy load.

■ *Use Wheels.* Use a dolly, wagon, or wheelbarrow whenever possible. Anything that requires noticeable effort to lift should be transported on wheels, even if it's just to take it to the other side of your workshop or garage.

■ *Push-Pull.* Let push come to shove! Pulling is more apt to jerk your back, so if you must: Push any carts, crates, and furniture with your back straight, knees and hips bent, and hands placed as close to shoulder height (to keep your back straight) as possible.

■ *Leaning Over and In.* For engine work, keep your back straight by bending at the hips and using one hand for support. Get a stool or tool box to stand on so you can position your feet and legs high enough to do a hip bend (*see Back Protection Principle #4, pg. 155*). Support your abdomen on the fender. Change positions about every 10 to 15 minutes. Stand up slowly and do pelvic tilts (*see Exercise #1, pg. 225*) or the standing back extension exercise (*see Exercise #6, pg. 234*) if you can do it comfortably.

■ *Work Bench.* Raise the surface of your work bench to 2 to 3 inches below elbow height. Leave room to place one foot under the work bench on a small stool, brick, or block, and leave enough room for both knees if your work requires sitting on a stool or chair.

■ *Overhead Storage and Shelves.* Store light objects on high shelves. Keep frequently used supplies and tools at bench height if possible. Have a sturdy ladder or portable steps that can be positioned so that you can get the light objects you need off of high shelves without twisting or leaning. Overhead light bulbs need changing, and a ladder for this "light" task is a bright idea.

CATS, DOGS, AND BACKS

If your back pain is severe, bedside petting—if you can reach your pet—is best. If your pain is moderate and the pet is small (cats and toy dogs), you probably are bending down to it, not lifting it up. If your pet is big (poodles and shepherds), it's leash walking (they can literally drag you down) that's apt to get you in the back. If it is a puppy, you probably ought to get someone to help, unless it has been house trained and is reasonably gentle. No matter what the size, you've got to feed and water your pet, clean up litter, and in the case of the latter, bigger is definitely not better.

- *Feeding.* Fill the food bowl on your kitchen counter and then kneel or squat to place it on the floor or on the ground. A large bowl can have food ladled or poured into it from a standing position. The bowl can be shoved into position with a cane, broom, or yardstick. The water bowl can be filled in similar fashion or replenished by a teapot, or via a small hose connected to a sink faucet.

- *Litter.* Litter can be swept into long-handled litter pans or picked up with a reacher-stick.

- *Cleaning and Grooming.* These should be done with care. All necessary equipment should be in place before starting, and it should be undertaken only if grooming can be completed in a short amount of time in order to avoid back strain.

22.

GETTING

BACK OUT

THE FIRST OUTING

A visit to the doctor is likely to be the first test for Severe Pain, Level 4 to Moderate Pain, Level 3. Plan to be a passenger if possible. If you are miserable, ask if there's a wheelchair available.

SHOPPING

■ *Severe Pain, Level 4 to Moderate Pain, Level 3.* Consider a taxi if you don't want to bother anyone. The driver can load and unload any of your packages. You have already invested a lot in your back, so a little additional cost for a cab to keep you on the mend may be more than justified. Plan to avoid rush-hour driving and crowded shopping center jostling. Plan for good parking. Plan to rest at home before taking in packages, or better, have someone else (the cab driver) bring them in for you. Take two shopping bags of your own with sturdy handles. You can pack one full shopping-bag load of purchases into two smaller bags for lighter and balanced load carrying. If the bottom drops out of a wet shopping bag, your back will probably drop out, too—so make sure your bags are water resistant.

- *Shopping Carts—Moderate Pain, Level 3.* Select a market with carts that have shallow baskets placed high on the cart, or bring your own cart. In any case, use wheels to save your back.

- *Loading—Moderate Pain, Level 3 to Mild Pain, Level 2.* Load the bags in the front or back seat of your car and not on the floor. The heaviest and most awkward package should be next to the door and easy to reach. If your car is a four-door model, place each bag on a seat next to a door. Hatchbacks are difficult and trunks are worse for loading and unloading. If you must use a trunk, use proper lifting techniques (*see Back Protection Principle #7, pg. 159*). Place your feet under the bumper or one leg on the bumper; or if you are tall and agile, one leg in the trunk when loading and unloading.

DEPARTMENT STORE—MODERATE PAIN, LEVEL 3

Pick a quiet time; plan for easy parking; avoid sales. Plan to rest when you get home. Choose a store that has a delivery service. Trying on clothes can be a trying experience on your back. Have the salesperson remove the clothes from the rack for you. Shop for loose-fitting, easily donned clothing. Twenty minutes of shopping is plenty your first time back out.

ELEVATOR—MODERATE PAIN, LEVEL 3 TO MILD PAIN, LEVEL 2

Stand back against the wall and flatten your back, keeping your knees and hips slightly flexed. Hold a pelvic tilt (*see Exercise #1, pg. 225*). Don't be afraid to tell others that you have a painful back. They'll appreciate knowing that and will want to help you.

BACK OUT FOR FUN

OUT TO DINNER—MODERATE PAIN, LEVEL 3 TO MILD PAIN, LEVEL 2

Pick a restaurant within a 20-minute driving radius. Be sure the parking is accessible. Make reservations so you will not have to stand or sit in an uncomfortable bar or hall waiting to be seated. Avoid booths. Pick a Back Seat. Have someone check out the seating if possible before you go to the restaurant. Let the owner or the maitre d' know you have a back problem. He's probably had one too and can be expected to be helpful.

Plan to eat light and order dishes that can be quickly prepared and quickly served. You don't want to linger over a prolonged, leisurely meal.

Take a portable back support, a firm purse, a rolled scarf, or a jacket to support the small of your back. If you forgot any of the above, ask the waiter for a tablecloth to roll or fold for a back support. Get up and walk around about every 20 minutes or so. The bathroom is a good place for some discreet wall slides (*see Exercise #19, pg. 253*) or back bends (*see Exercise #6, pg. 234*).

THE THEATER: BACK TO SHOW BIZ—MODERATE PAIN, LEVEL 3 TO MILD PAIN, LEVEL 2

The basic outing problems—close proximity for parking (let someone drop you off at the entrance) and good seating—are similar to going to a restaurant. Unique to a theater are aisles, balconies, escalators (barrier-free elevators), and intermissions.

Seating, as always, must be carefully selected, as few theaters have comfortable seats. Take along a portable seat support, a firm padded purse, a rolled jacket or towel, or a pillow for back support. When it comes to seating, *know your show before you go*. In fact, you should plan for some standing during the show by choosing an aisle seat. Not only will this keep you from climbing over or being climbed on by others, but you can stretch your legs more readily and leave without disturbing others if need be. About every 20 to 30 minutes you may want to stand up and walk about, or stand against the wall and do some pelvic tilts, wall slides, or back bends to relieve the stiffness in your back. If you are starting to feel tired or achy, leave at intermission, or even sooner if need be. Whenever you do leave, wait until the crowd thins before you make your exit. No applause is better than being clapped *back* in bed.

BACK IN THE PARK—MODERATE PAIN, LEVEL 3 TO MILD PAIN, LEVEL 2

Parking in the park can be a problem. Try a weekday or early morning for your first time out. Park benches are so-so for sitting, but can function fairly well as a makeshift bed—and it's all too obvious how many are being used for just that purpose.

It's sitting without a good back support that's a major problem in the park. Folding chairs have a huge gap just where your back needs support, and so do most bench seats at the park. Canvas folding backrests are also poor providers of back support, so you really have to plan to lie down unless you are lucky enough to find a portable bench seat that hits you just right.

BACK IN THE BALLPARK—MODERATE PAIN, LEVEL 3 TO MILD PAIN, LEVEL 2

Lest the first crack of the bat be a crack in your back—it's important to think about problems at the ball park or stadium. Parking, long walks, long lines, long aisles, long stair climbs, poor seating, and jostling crowds are likely if it's a game worth watching. If it isn't—you still have long walks, long aisles, long stairs, and poor back seating (no matter what you pay for admission).

If you know you can negotiate the walk and steps, then be sure you've taken along enough back support paraphernalia to make a Back Seat. This may include a real or makeshift footstool as well, to keep your feet from dangling and adding a strain to your back. If you've got this all together—okay, play ball!

BACK IN THE WORLD: TRAVEL

If you're at Severe Pain, Level 4 or Moderate Pain, Level 3, you're not ready for the grand tour, or even a local commuter flight. If you're at Moderate Pain, Level 3 (and you have to go) or Mild Pain, Level 2 (and you're ready to go), the suggestions in Chapter 17 will give you useful tips to keep you on the go.

23.

BACK IN LOVE

"Not tonight dear, I have a headache—or a backache" can either be a classic psychological withholding manipulation or a sincere and appropriate painful response to equally sincere amorous approaches.

SEX, ROMANCE, AND LOVE

Sex is a universal biological experience, essential to all beings. It is a source of pleasure, is essential to procreation, and for many is the basis for parenting. *Love* may be as universal, but is less apparent in many species. *Romance*, like the courtship dances of insects, reptiles, birds, and humans, is certainly stimulating to all kinds of critters, poets, and fools—like you and me. If sex is an act that can be a source of great pleasure even in the absence of love, and love is the sublime expression of affection, then romance is the catalyst that heightens the expression of love and can lead to its ultimate, physically and spiritually fulfilling expression in sexual relations. Romance can also lead to soaring fantasies and crushing disappointments when love and the performance of sex fail to meet expectations.

So what has this to do with low back pain? If you have low back pain, you have to reestablish your priorities to get well, function, and stay well. Since love and sex are universal phenomena, loving (even grandma bending over to fondle the grandchild) and sex must be given a priority and the opportunity to flower.

BACK TO BASICS

If you want sex but are in pain, or you are unsure just how well your back will hold up during sex—you need guidance.

If your low back pain is Severe Pain, Level 4, stay with love and gentle romance. Closeness, tenderness (write letters, phone, or send flowers), kissing, and caressing are all expressions of love and are appropriate, but attempts at more active sex may prove impossible. Masturbation, if socially and culturally acceptable, may be the most practical means of sexual pleasuring.

If your low back pain is Moderate Pain, Level 3, a little more romance is possible. There is never too much love, but sex needs some planning.

PAIN

Medications, such as narcotics and tranquilizers, and muscle relaxants like alcohol may inhibit male potency and female desire. It is best to experiment with medications for pain in advance if disappointment is to be avoided.

PLANNING

Arrange for successful sex. Rest to avoid fatigue, and schedule a painless day so your back will not be in knots at the time you and your partner have planned for sex. Have lots of pillows handy to help you adjust for positions of comfort and pleasure. A warm bath may be soothing and your body will probably be more inviting if you choose that over a cold pack for pain control.

PLEASURE

Enjoy lots of foreplay stimulation (this may shorten the actual sexual intercourse but not the pleasure) and, when desired, masturbation, particularly if sexual intercourse proves uncomfortable. During intercourse, use smooth, slow, sensuous movements, and if you are a natural athlete in bed, wait until you are in better condition—consider your initial efforts as "spring training." Learn and gently explore each other's anatomy. Be rewarded by discovery. Here again, it's hard to discard previously established moral precepts—and if sexual participation is fraught with guilt, it's best avoided. There *is* life after sex.

POSITIONS

The best guide to back comfort during sex is to accommodate the positions you have already found comfortable for your back, and creatively adapt them to the sex act. Remember, if you have a tennis elbow, you may have to run around your back-hand to stay in the game. So, do whatever works to get *back in love*.

The pelvic tilt (*see Exercise #1, pg. 225*) is the key position for back protection and pleasure. The pelvic tilt exercise is basic to the sex act, and a slow, gentle pelvic tilt while thrusting can be very therapeutic.

The next most important consideration is that you ask your partner to keep as much of his or her weight off of you as possible. This generally means that if it is your back that is aching and your partner can support his or her weight, you will want your back to be on the bed.

A third rule is that the partner with the healthy back becomes the major thrustor and the *back in lover* the principal thrustee in the partnership.

Options to consider:
1. You are supine or semi-reclining, with a pillow under your buttocks and another small pillow beneath the small of your back, in a back-flat position. Your partner should be kneeling and straddling above you (*see Fig. 14*).

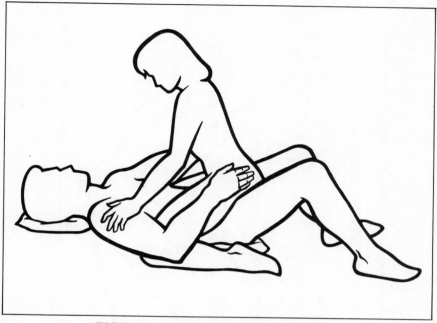

FIGURE 14 THE STRADDLE POSITION

2. You are side-lying with your lower leg slightly flexed, and penetration can be from the front or the rear (*see Fig. 15*).
3. You are seated in a chair with your foot or feet on a stool, and your partner straddles in front of you front-to-front, or you can be seated front-to-back in a rocking chair, again with a foot on the stool. The latter position only works if the male partner is the one with back problems and is able to penetrate from behind. In all these postures, every effort is made to keep your back as flat as possible or slightly rounded in a pelvic tilt.

THE BACK-OFF CAUTION SIGNAL

It is a good idea to have an agreed-upon signal to indicate that pain is beginning, in order to prevent further discomfort and possibly the discouragement of future relations. It's equally desirous in all lovemaking to let each other know what caresses and stimuli are most enhancing to the act.

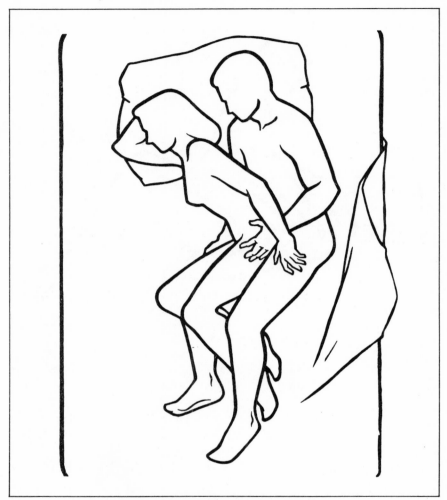

FIGURE 15 THE SPOON POSITION

ALTERNATIVE STIMULI

(If there are no social, cultural, or personal barriers.) When sexual intercourse is not feasible, oral stimuli by licking, sucking, or mechanical vibration may provide an important basis for mutual stimulation and caressing.

If your low back pain is Mild Pain, Level 2, you can use any of the above options or strategies to enhance your sexual pleasure. Overly robust sexual activity may cause discomfort, but it's highly unlikely that lovemaking will result in significant harm to your back. *If your low back pain is Minimal Pain, Level 1*, then you're probably like all of the rest of us, and if you are having problems with sex, it's almost sure that it is not your back that is causing the problem. Nonetheless, since sexual dysfunction, regardless of its cause, is a serious disability, it is essential that we put any sexual dysfunction into proper perspective.

PERSPECTIVES

Perspectives on why "not tonight, dear."—Sex, love, and romance are all interrelated, yet each can exist in the absence of the others. Witness rape, unrequited love, and romantic dreams. Sexual failure can result from a lack of romance, opportunity, or love. The "not tonight" may be an excuse for avoiding an unpleasant act. It may be a manifestation of depression and represent a lack or loss of self-esteem. It may be an expression of concern about pregnancy, or a worry about causing harm to one's partner who has pain or other illness.

A lack of or decrease in sexual activity can produce debilitating emotional stress. A person's perception of himself or herself as one who is not only capable of but entitled to enjoying love, caressing, and sexual interaction, is a crucial component of his or her whole psychic and physiological being. For some people, there is life after sex. But for others, the sense of not being sexually active or desirable can be insidiously and terribly crushing. In our culture it often seems that people who are crippled, in pain, ill, aged, fat, or thin are considered undesirable by many as objects of sex. This is a great tragedy and an unfortunate reflection of our societal immaturity and insensitivity. For the individual so-stigmatized, psychological counseling may help restore self-confidence, self-worth, and the courage to be loved.

Finally, the ability to have or sustain an erection is crucial to consummation of the act of intercourse, but not to love and romance. Failure of erection or desire is very, very rarely the result of disk-related problems. (*See "Spinal Stenosis," pg. 31*). The point is that if your sex life is not what it should be, it may have nothing to do with your back or medications. Counseling with your physician and possibly with a sex counselor or psychiatrist may well be in order.

24.

BACK TO WORK

In the house, garden, garage, and work place, the same principles always apply. The Four Back Words (*see pg. 63*) are still
fore-most. *Pacing* the work; flexing and stretching frequently to
avoid muscle tension; and *facing* the work whenever picking up,
reaching, or lowering are important rules (*see* Feet First and
Face It!, *pg. 150*). You pace the work to avoid fatigue from
overuse or prolonged fixed postures (e.g., searching for papers in
the lower file drawer can eventually cause back strain). Flex to
relieve muscle strain by doing five to ten pelvic tilts (*see Exercise
#1, pg. 225*) or wall slides (*see Exercise #10, pg. 239*) and, if
tolerated, five to ten standing back bends (*see Exercise #6, pg.
234*) every 20 minutes. Facing the work means that you pivot to
change positions or directions (if seated, you use a swivel chair) in
order to move with your feet first and avoid twisting your back.
Let's *face it—feet first!*

LIGHT WORK

MOSTLY STANDING

These are jobs such as salesperson, supervisor, security patrol, surgeon, machine operator, and clerks.

■ *Shoes*. Good shoes give you a key to *under-standing*. A good shoe is well fitted with no more than a 1″ heel and has rubber soles and heels for shock absorption. If arch supports are recommended, they should preferably be custom-made. If your foot aches, an appropriate custom *orthosis* may be required so that the muscle tension in your legs due to foot strain does not also cause back muscle tension and increased back pain.

■ *The Floor*. A rubber mat or wood grill can relieve the strain of prolonged standing on hard surfaces. A low stool or footrail will permit posture change and minimize strain. Tired feet can lead to back strain—so it's important to have a proper *under-standing* for your feet.

■ *Standing with Frequent Bending*. Keep your back flat and straight, but not necessarily vertical. Bend from the hips. Your feet should be about a shoulder's width apart with your knees relaxed, slightly bent, and definitely not locked. Change leg position by using a stepstool, and stretch by doing pelvic tilts, squats, and especially back bends (*see Chapter 26*) if they are comfortable for you. These should be done five to ten times and at intervals frequent enough to avoid muscle fatigue and back strain. Use your arms for added support.

■ *Work Surface*. The bench top or counter should be approximately 2 to 3 inches below your elbow height when standing. If you have to hunch your shoulders up to work, you know your work surface is too high.

■ *Surface Inclination*. This should ideally be a 10 to 15 degree slope up and away from you for easy access, unless a level surface is essential to avoid spilling or for other technical reasons.

■ *Tools and Supplies*. Arrange for frequently used equipment to be within easy grasp. Store heavy objects at table or counter height and within easy reach—preferably accessible for sliding rather than lifting. Store only small, light objects on high shelves.

■ *Reaching Across Counters or Up.* Face the object feet first. Place one foot forward and reach with the hand on the same side to grasp the object. Support yourself by putting the opposite hand on the counter, or lift with both hands if the object is heavy.

■ *Switches, Controls, and Pedals.* These devices should be within easy reach and easy to manipulate.

■ *Occasionally Carrying a Heavy Load.* This concerns service trades with tools, sales with samples, students with books, waitresses with trays, and building trades with tools and equipment. Whenever possible, divide heavy, bulky loads into two smaller parcels and balance the loads with one in each hand, or better, make two trips. Keep your arms close to your body when lifting. Use handles whenever possible and *face it—feet first!*

MOSTLY KNEELING—CARPET LAYING, TILE SETTING, FLOORING

The techniques for "The Garden" (*see Chapter 21*) apply here. Pacing and frequent breaks, for stretching to prevent prolonged postural strain, are important. Use knee pads to minimize knee strain. Bend at the hips. Raise the buttocks and keep the back flat or slightly arched inwardly (swaybacked), never rounded. When reaching out, use the opposite hand to support your weight again, taking the bend in the hips and knees.

MOSTLY SITTING—SECRETARIES, RECEPTIONISTS, ASSEMBLERS, TECHNICIANS, PHYSICIANS, EXECUTIVES

All should take a Back Seat (*see Chapter 18*). Wear glasses if you need them, and have adequate soft lighting to prevent eye, neck, and back strain. Arrange for your telephone, typewriter, terminal, and files to be accessible and at a comfortable height. There should be adequate knee room under the desk so that you can sit close to your work. A small footstool helps support your feet and allows for a comfortable leg position change.

Keep frequently used items in close proximity to avoid overreaching (e.g., telephone, writing supplies). Store items at a comfortable level to minimize overhead reaching, or bending to lower drawers and shelves. Use desktop trays, adjoining desk files, or credenzas to promote efficiency and back protection. Remember—*Feet First and Face It!* Prop up papers or reading and reference materials to reduce leaning forward, thus promoting good head, neck, and back posture. Propping suggestions include: standing clip boards, magnetic paper holders, dense foam wedges, or large, empty three-ring binders (closed on the desk). Book holders can reduce postural stresses on the neck, shoulders, arms, and back when reading. If necessary, you can create an angled desk surface by placing blocks under the rear legs of the desk or by purchasing a desk top with a tilt mechanism (i.e., a drafting table). Table edging serves as a ledge to keep paper or pencils from slipping off the edge of a tilted desk.

Check your chair to see that it moves easily. Try a Lucite or plastic mat on the floor for greater ease of movement. Be sure your casters are appropriate for the flooring beneath you. Soft casters are for hard surfaces and hard casters are for soft carpeted surfaces.

Evaluate your telephone work habits. A built-up phone handle, a speaker phone, or a headset can eliminate prolonged holding of the phone. Maintain good head, neck, and back posture while phoning, and avoid cradling the phone in your neck.

DIFFICULT SEATING

Analyze your work situation and correct as many problems as possible.

■ *Dentists, Hygienists, Beauticians, Barbers, and Surgeons.* There are unavoidable cramped postures in the dental profession as well as in many service, repair, and technical jobs. Flexibility in seat and work-level adjustment, along with frequent position changes and stretches, will keep your back limber and minimize strain.

If possible, get up and walk around every 15 to 20 minutes. Do some wall slides (*see Exercise #19, pg. 253*) and back bends (*see Exercise #6, pg. 234*). While seated, try to maintain a Seated Tripod posture (*see Fig. 12, pg. 167*) with your back straight. Whenever you can, rock slowly back and forth over your ischial tuberosities. First, rotate the pelvis backward as in a seated pelvic tilt, and then arch the back (swayback) by rotating the pelvis forward. This will keep the back from getting stiff and aching from holding a cramped position for too long.

■ *Computer Terminal Operators.* Eyestrain and neck and back strain are common hazards. The screen on your computer should be adjustable as to its height and angle and intensity of light. In general, the screen should be placed so that if you are looking straight ahead you are looking at the top of the screen. The screen should be positioned about 18 to 20 inches away from your eyes. The keyboard should be low enough so that your arms can hang freely and so that your elbows are bent at right angles. Detachable keyboards and split-level desk designs are ideal for this. Wrist support bars are also available to help rest your arms and thereby minimize back strain. The computer should be placed on a table at a height of 25 to 29 inches. Adjust the height of the work table or desk as necessary so that your legs can easily be placed beneath it. Your arms should be positioned close to your body to increase control, decrease fatigue, and promote maintenance of proper posture. Take a Back Seat.

■ *Dental Patient.* That's you! Even if you are just having your teeth cleaned, the dental chair is a *back* trap. Explain your problem to the dentist and hygienist so they can adjust the chair and ease your back. This is particularly true in rinsing and spitting during procedures. If your back problem is *severe* (Pain Level 4) or *moderately severe* (Pain Level 3) and your dental problem is not, wait until your back is better before you open your mouth. The same type of problem can also arise at the *hairdresser* and the *barber* (especially when your hair is being washed) and even in the doctor's office—so let them know your problem and help them find the best solutions.

MOSTLY DRIVING—TRUCK DRIVERS, TAXICAB DRIVERS,
SALESPERSONS, PILOTS, CAR POOLERS, AND YOU

Let's face it—most of us spend a lot of time in a car. Some get paid for driving. Others either don't get paid unless they drive to work, or have to pay someone else to chauffeur their kids. All the rules for "Take a Back Seat" (*see Chapter 18*) apply. So don't fasten your seatbelt for a long haul until you are sure the seat is right, or at least that you have made it right with pillows, cushions, and back supports. Power steering, power brakes, automatic transmission, and cruise control are all important features in minimizing back strain. If you're going to be driving, and you have a choice, choose a car with a Back Seat and power-assisted controls.

MODERATE AND HEAVY WORK

The basic rules all apply. The tips for garage and workshop on one- and two-man lifting, with emphasis on smooth, coordinated moves (synchronize hip, hand, and knee bend) and foot-first pivots are especially important. Vary the tasks as much as possible to avoid fatigue from prolonged repetition or heavy lifting. Push rather than pull if possible. Use good tools and keep them in good working order—they are easier to repair than your back.

V.

EXERCISE,

FITNESS, AND

FUN

25.

BACK RECONDITIONING:

FEEL GOOD,

DO GOOD,

BE GOOD

Exercises are the active components of back pain treatment. There are exercises that can be right for you even if you have severe back pain.

Exercises can help to relieve pain, and at The Arthritis & Back Pain Center, we call these the "Feel-Good" Easing Exercises. They should feel good! If not, you may be performing them incorrectly, or they may not be right for you, so check with your doctor or physical therapist before proceeding further. The same admonition applies to exercises that stretch, strengthen, and recondition your back. You may feel a good, hard stretch, but you should feel no aggravation of your back symptoms while you are doing your exercises or afterward. These reconditioning or "Do-Good" Exercises should do just that—good, not harm—so read on, and learn how to get a bad back into good shape.

EXERCISE—WHEN IS IT SUPPOSED TO HURT?

There are definitely different strokes for different folks, and having low back pain may be the only thing folks have in common. Some of us are convinced that if exercise does not hurt (as in the case of medicine, when it doesn't taste bad), it can't do any good. Others feel that any discomfort caused during or after exercise means that it is harmful. How do we distinguish between the level of discomfort or hurt that is desirable, or at least unavoidable, during exercise and a *hurt that means harm*?

Any exercise, including all of those illustrated in this book, can cause pain if it is not appropriate to your problem, or if it is not properly executed. If you are in doubt about the effects of any exercise, don't try it, and if you've been doing it, stop and seek a professional opinion from your physician or therapist.

"Feel-Good" Easing Exercises should all feel comfortable and become more comfortable with each repetition, as they are designed to give relief by gently stretching tight muscles. Nonetheless, the comfortable feeling associated with doing the exercise may be accompanied by a stretching sensation that is worrisome.

THE HEALTHY-STRETCH PAIN TEST

To distinguish an acceptable level of discomfort during a stretching exercise from a potentially aggravating pain, you can perform the following tests:

1. Perform Exercise #12, (*see pg. 242*). Use the "good" leg for this test if you have sciatic pain.
2. When you feel a mild pulling or tight sensation behind your knee, bend your foot and toes toward you as far as you can and continue to stretch. This will cause a decided burning, stretching discomfort in the back of your leg as long as you maintain the stretch. None of your exercises should hurt more than this, and in fact, they should cause less discomfort. When you are doing your exercises properly, you should feel the stretch in the area indicated by the symbol on your exercise illustration (*see Fig. 16, pg. 225*). Or, a muscle fatigue-strain will be felt in the muscles to be strengthened, also marked by a symbol.

Anytime you begin a new exercise, you can expect some new discomfort or mild achiness after the first few sessions as your muscles adapt to unaccustomed activity—you probably know this from past experience when you resume any sport at the start of the season. Never force an exercise. If it's a stretch—let it stretch. All exercises should be smoothly executed without jerks, bounces, or plops. You can relax better if you breath in and out slowly with your mouth open while you are stretching. Seduce your muscles—don't assault them! If it's a muscle-strengthening exercise, hold or tense only the muscles involved. Avoid straining your neck during any abdomen-strengthening exercise. If the exercise aggravates your usual back pain while you're doing it or causes an increase of your customary pain on the following day, you may be doing something wrong. Try it again more gently the next time, making as sure as possible that you are following instructions correctly; better yet, get a professional opinion from your physician or therapist.

"FEEL-GOOD" EASING EXERCISES

The "Feel-Good" Easing Exercises on pg. 263 are basic stretches that you can try. They often provide some immediate relief to back pain. These exercises (with the exception of the Knee Back Exercises #7 and #8 on pp. 235, 236) are also important to the back reconditioning process.

"DO-GOOD" BACK RECONDITIONING EXERCISES

The three major components of low back pain management are:

1. Learning to prevent pain by the use of proper body mechanics.

2. Relieving pain by medicine, therapy, and "Feel-Good" Easing Exercises.

3. Increasing strength, resiliency, and tolerance for body activities by muscle conditioning—what we call *"Do-Good"* Exercises.

HOW DO "DO-GOOD" EXERCISES DO GOOD?

In contrast to the immediate benefits of "Feel-Good" Easing Exercises, "Do-Good" Exercises take *time* to do good. If you've been in pain for more than a few days, your muscles can become tight and lose their strength; and after a few weeks, there's inevitable deterioration of muscle strength and tightening and shortening of the adjacent connecting tissues.

The first objective of "Do-Good" Exercises is to begin stretching to relieve muscle spasms and permit better alignment of skeletal structures. The next objective is to restore strength to the muscles that support your back or that permit you to move without straining your back. When you've had a back pain episode and are now on the mend, you'll want to get back to normal activities as soon as possible. But what was normal before is not normal now—because your back has become deconditioned. If you attempt your customary routine without proper reconditioning, you could expect a setback. No pitcher expects to start the season and pitch nine innings without several months of spring training. He and his coach know he'll be out of action for most of the season with a sore arm if he tries. Your back can be out for "the season" too if you don't provide it with proper pre-season "Do-Good" Exercise conditioning.

DO GOOD ONE STEP AT A TIME

Just doing a therapeutic exercise once doesn't mean you've had the benefit of it. A marathon runner has to start running short distances and build his endurance. A weight lifter works out with light weights and gradually progresses to heavy ones.

Your exercise program should start with simple basic exercises and build gradually to more vigorous and demanding conditioning. Allow time for muscles to become strong and for tight tissues to gradually stretch out.

GUIDELINES FOR RECONDITIONING EXERCISE

Start with Exercise #1, the Basic Pelvic Tilt (*see pg. 225*). Be sure that you can do it as prescribed without problems, once a day on Day 1, and then twice a day on Day 2. Then add the next exercise, #2, Single Knee to Chest (*see pg. 227*) and proceed further in the same manner. Don't try to rush back to health by doing two or more new exercises at a time. If five repetitions[5]

---

[5]A repetition for any exercise consists of moving from the starting position, through the exercise, and returning to the starting position. This is one repetition.

twice a day is right—fifty repetitions ten times a day is *not*. Settle back. Give nature a chance—don't try to blast your way *back* to health. By giving a couple of days' time before initiating a new exercise, you have a chance to observe any untoward effects from the previous exercise before proceeding further. Listen to your body and pay particular attention to *back* talk.

If your symptoms are subsiding, add one exercise every two to three days. *If your back pain is worse,* back up a little. Stop the most recent exercise and do the preceding one more gently. Consider whether the worsening is due to something you are doing during the day or to the latest exercise—you have already established that you can tolerate the previous ones.

HOW LONG BEFORE I'M READY TO GET BACK TO NORMAL?

If your back pain is Severe Pain, Level 4 or Moderate Pain, Level 3, and has lasted a week or less, you should wait three weeks (while doing daily exercises progressing up to your achievable pain level). If your back pain has lasted longer than one week, add two weeks of "Do-Good" Exercises for each week of pain, or eight additional weeks of conditioning after you have improved to the Mild Pain, Level 2 or Minimal Pain, Level 1 stage. Once you have reached your conditioning goal and have maintained your exercises at your best level on a twice-daily basis for two to four weeks, you're ready to cut back to your long-term maintenance program (*see Chapter 27*). If there is one classic *back* trap, it's the "gee, I feel good today, I think I'll catch up on everything" decision. Housecleaning, chores, hikes, long rides, the theater, a set of tennis, or exercise class—take any three of these on your first good day and the next day will be a bad one. Reconditioning takes time—take the time to get well.

26.

"DO-GOOD"

BACK RECONDITIONING

EXERCISES

The twenty-five carefully illustrated and carefully worded exercises in this chapter have provided the core of The Arthritis & Back Pain Center's low back pain treatment program. There are exercises for each level of back pain with cautions about any problems you may experience when trying them.

It is important that you understand what each exercise is designed to do for you so that you can appreciate its significance and perform it effectively. To help you gain understanding, we have provided four symbols: strengthening, stretching, direction of movement in the back-bend exercises, and direction of movement in the knee back and rotation exercises. The symbols are placed over the muscles to be strengthened or stretched. You will see that certain exercises (Exercise #1, #17, #22, and #23) may stretch or strengthen more than one muscle group, or as in the case of Exercise #1, may stretch the low back and buttocks muscles while strengthening the abdominal muscles.

The exercises are numbered in the order in which they are best tolerated and best utilized. Exercises #1–#4 and #5–#8 can be used for Severe Pain, Level 4; Exercises #9–#14 are used for Moderate Pain, Level 3; Exercises #15–#23 for Mild Pain, Level

2; and Exercises #24 and #25 can be added for Minimal Pain, Level 1. In Minimal Pain, Level 1, specific conditioning for various athletic activities can be added; then you will be ready for a maintenance program and conditioning.

In addition, certain exercises have been developed that not only add to the back reconditioning therapy and help prevent pain, but also actually help relieve pain. These are the "Feel-Good" Easing Exercises that are a part of our exercise series, and they are listed on pg. 263.

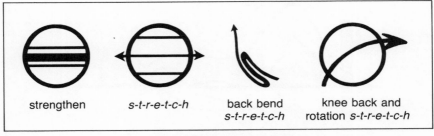

strengthen   *s-t-r-e-t-c-h*   back bend *s-t-r-e-t-c-h*   knee back and rotation *s-t-r-e-t-c-h*

FIGURE 16 EXERCISE SYMBOLS

SEVERE PAIN, LEVEL 4 CONDITIONING EXERCISES

#1 BASIC PELVIC TILT

This exercise is the basis for all back conditioning and back protection postures. It should be initiated as soon as pain permits. A milder form of this exercise—consisting of a mild buttock or anal squeeze or pinch—should be used before each of the exercises and before changing position or commencing new activities, or to help relieve back tension during prolonged standing, sitting, or kneeling.

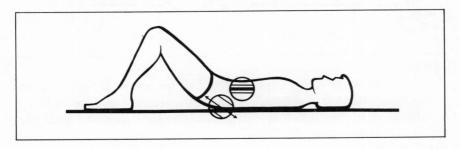

PURPOSE: Generally, to relieve discomfort associated with back pain.

More specifically:

1. to *s-t-r-e-t-c-h* the low back (*lumbosacral spine*) and the hips;

2. to begin strengthening the abdominal and buttock (*gluteal*) muscles.

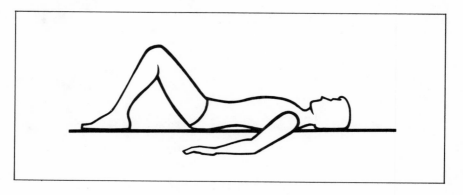

METHOD:

1. Lie on your back on a firm flat surface or on the floor (*if you can get up easily*). Bend your knees. Rest your feet *flat* on the "floor." (*A small pillow may be used under your head for comfort.*)

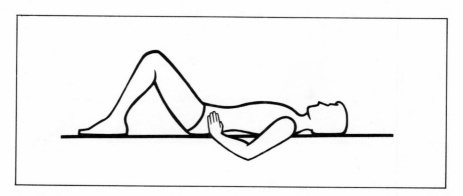

2. Place your fingers on the front of the crest of your pelvis.

3. Squeeze your buttocks tightly together (*imagine holding a coin between the buttocks*). This flattens the back and initiates the pelvic tilt.

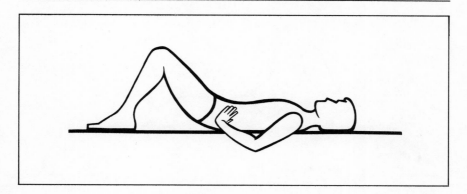

4. Now tighten the abdominal muscles to complete the pelvic tilt. You should feel your fingers moving backwards as your pelvis is tilting to flatten and *s-t-r-e-t-c-h* your lower back.

5. Hold this *tilted* position. *Do not hold your breath.* Count out loud from 1001 to 1006.

6. Relax.

7. Repeat three to five times, once or twice hourly during the day when in bed, and at least twice daily during convalescence.

#2 SINGLE KNEE TO CHEST

This exercise stretches the low back and the muscles of the buttocks in a gentle fashion, one leg at a time.

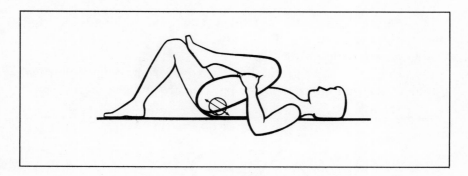

PURPOSE: Generally, to relieve discomfort associated with back pain.

More specifically: to *s-t-r-e-t-c-h* the low back (*lumbosacral*) and the buttock (*gluteal*) muscles.

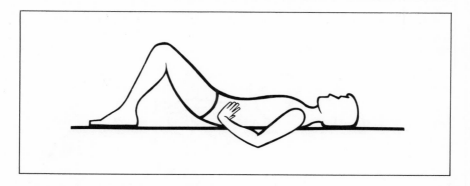

METHOD:

1. Lie on your back on a firm flat surface or on the floor. Bend your knees. Rest your feet *flat* on the "floor." (*A small pillow may be used under your head for comfort.*)

2. Do a mild pelvic tilt.

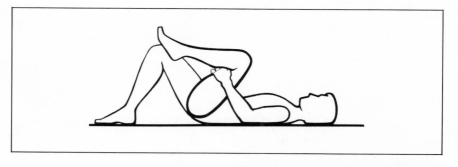

3. Slowly, raise your *left* knee. Grasp just behind your left knee with both hands.

4. Release the pelvic tilt.

5. Pull your knee gradually toward your chest until you feel a mild s-t-r-e-t-c-h in your lower back or at the back of your hip.

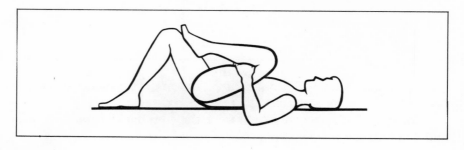

6. Hold position and count out loud: 1001, 1002, and 1003. DO NOT HOLD YOUR BREATH.

7. Relax.

8. Repeat the pelvic tilt. Keep your knee bent and slowly return your foot to the starting position.

9. Repeat the exercise by slowly pulling your *right* knee toward your chest until you again feel the *s-t-r-e-t-c-h* in your lower back or at the back of your hip.

10. Repeat three to five times, twice daily until you're on a maintenance program. If the exercise relieves back pain, three to five repetitions can be done once or twice hourly for pain control.

#3 PARTIAL "SIT-UP" (ABDOMINAL ISOMETRIC)

This exercise helps strengthen the abdominal wall, and since your abdominal wall is nature's own corset, this exercise is extremely important for back pain protection. When you can hold the partial "sit-up" for 40 seconds, you should be able to go about your usual daily activities without a corset or brace. Your abdominal muscles are strong enough to support you unless you have a special problem that requires continuous bracing.

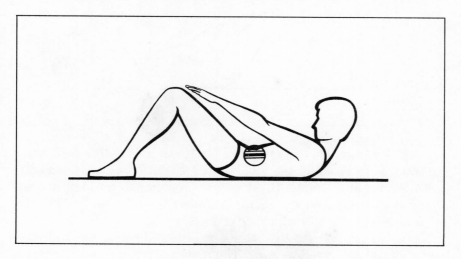

PURPOSE: to strengthen the abdominal muscles in order to help alleviate stress on the back muscles.

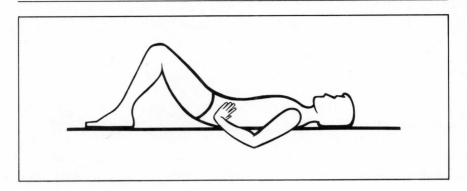

METHOD:

1. Lie on your back on a firm flat surface or on the floor. Bend your knees. Rest your feet *flat* on the "floor." (*A small pillow may be used under your head for comfort.*)

2. Do a mild pelvic tilt. If possible, hold the tilt throughout the exercise.

3. Keep your chin *tucked in* and use your abdominal muscles to slowly lift your head and shoulders as you reach your hands as close as possible to your knees. Breathe out as you sit up. DO NOT GRASP YOUR KNEES.

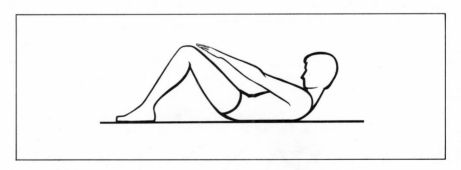

4. Initially, hold the position for 10 seconds and repeat twice, gradually increasing the holding time until you can hold the position for 40 seconds. Be sure your abdominal muscles, and not your neck, help you reach. DO NOT HOLD YOUR BREATH. Breathe in and out slowly during this exercise.

5. Return slowly to starting position. Jerking up and plopping back, as one does in a conventional sit-up, is potentially dangerous in any exercise, including the partial sit-up.

6. Relax.

7. Repeat twice daily until you're on a maintenance program.

#4 KNEE PUSH WITH CHAIR
(ALTERNATE ABDOMINAL ISOMETRIC)

This exercise can be substituted for the Partial "Sit-Up" when neck or leg pain is a problem.

PURPOSE: to strengthen the abdominal muscles, which will decrease stress on the lower back.

METHOD:
1. Lie on your back with your knees bent and your feet placed beneath a chair.
2. Do a mild pelvic tilt.

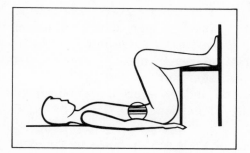

3. Slowly place the leg of your most painful side on the seat of the chair. Follow with your opposite leg.
4. Keeping your upper arms flat on the floor and your elbows slightly bent, place your hands on your thighs.

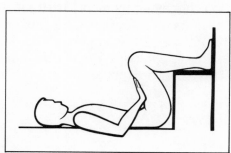

5. Do a *forceful* pelvic tilt as you push with your hands against your thighs. Resist the hand-pressure with your thighs.
6. Hold position and count out loud: from 1001 to 1006. DO NOT HOLD YOUR BREATH. Try to push harder with each count.
7. Relax.

8. Slowly return your foot on the most painful side, and then your opposite foot, to the starting position.

9. Repeat ten times, two times per day; or hold for a count of 40, two times per day.

SPECIAL PAIN CONTROL EXERCISES (#5–#8)

Conventional wisdom has cautioned for years against leaning backward if you have a low back pain or a sciatic pain. It is now recognized that many patients will benefit from a slow repetitive back bend if it can be done without pinching the sciatic nerve or straining the small facet joints in the lower back. The concept is that leaning back squeezes gooey bulging disk material forward away from the bulge. This can relieve pain or back strain and help prevent recurrences for moderate to minimal pain levels if done before and after strenuous or prolonged exercise or activity (such as gardening), or inactivity (such as long drive or watching TV). Do these exercises *only if you have first been evaluated by your doctor*, specifically taught the correct method, and can perform the exercises without increasing pain.

The Knee Back exercises (#7 and #8) were designed for low back pain sufferers by Dr. Alec Thompson, D.O. These exercises can be helpful in relieving aching or persistent pain in the low back or buttocks. Whether or not the exercise helps by relieving sacroiliac strain, as Dr. Thompson suggested, is moot, but that it often provides some relief is certainly true. The Knee Back exercise can be performed lying or sitting. It is important to be relaxed when performing the exercise. Exercise #8 can be done while sitting at work or while traveling, as a means of relieving discomfort.

#5 PRESS-UPS

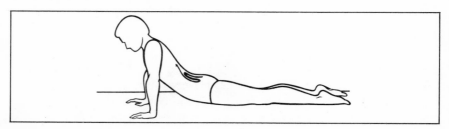

PURPOSE:

1. to return disk material to its proper position and move it away from pain-sensitive nerves;

2. to provide a backward s-t-r-e-t-c-h to maintain spinal mobility.

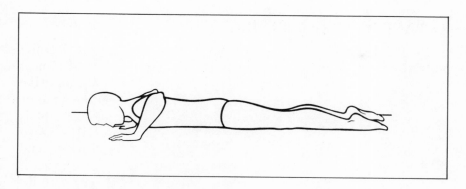

METHOD:

1. Lie flat on your stomach with the palms of your hands under your shoulders.

2. Relax your back, buttocks, and legs. Have your legs slightly apart.

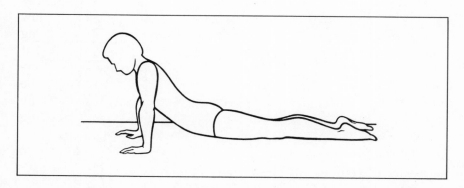

3. Keep your hips on the floor and your chin tucked in as you straighten your arms in a steady, controlled manner.

4. DO NOT HOLD THIS POSITION. Return to the starting position smoothly.

5. Count as you repeat movement: "Up, 2, 3, and down, 2, 3." Remember: DO NOT HOLD THE "UP" POSITION.

6. Repeat ten times, once or twice hourly for pain relief, and

five to ten times before, during, and after strenuous or sustained
activities or before and after your regular exercises.

Caution: Stop the exercise if pain increases in the buttocks
or legs.

#6 BACK BENDS, STANDING

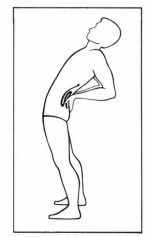

PURPOSE: to squeeze viscous disk material forward and away from the pain-sensitive
area.

METHOD:
1. Stand in a straight-back posture with
your feet a shoulder's width apart.

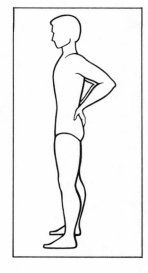

2. Place your hands at waist level on
each side of your back. Allow your thumbs
to wrap around to the front and your fingers to lie over your low back.

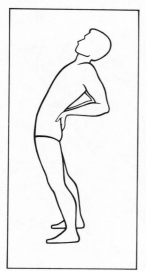

3. Keeping your knees straight and maintaining a chin-tucked position, relax your back and bend back at the waist; then return to the straight-posture position. DO NOT COME FORWARD PAST THE STRAIGHT-BACK POSTURE.

4. In a steady, controlled manner, bend back, saying, "Pres-sure on, pres-sure off," as you repeat the movement.

5. Repeat ten times, once or twice hourly for pain relief, and five to ten times before, during, and after strenuous or sustained activities or before and after your regular exercises.

Caution: Stop the exercise if pain increases in your legs or buttocks.

#7 KNEE BACK (LYING)

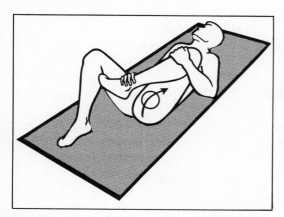

PURPOSE: to relieve pain radiating into the buttock by gently s-t-r-e-t-c-h-i-n-g tense buttock (*gluteal*) muscles.

METHOD:

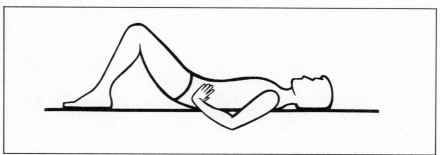

1. Lie down and do a gentle pelvic tilt.

2. Move your left knee toward your left elbow.

3. Relax the pelvic tilt.

4. Grasp your left ankle with your right hand, keeping your elbows away from your side.

5. Place your left hand on the front of your left leg below the knee.

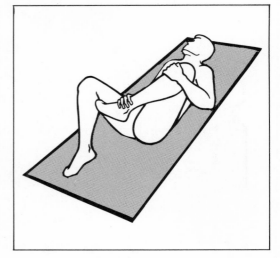

6. Gently press your heel toward your groin and, *at the same time*, gently pull your knee toward the left elbow.

7. Hold this position and count from 1001 to 1010. The count may be increased to 1020.

8. Repeat the exercise on the opposite side.

9. Repeat three to five times, once or twice each hour as long as pain relief is being obtained.

Caution: Stop the exercise if pain increases or if numbness or tingling occurs.

#8 KNEE BACK (SITTING)

PURPOSE: to relieve pain radiating into the buttocks by *s-t-r-e-t-c-h-i-n-g* tense buttock muscles.

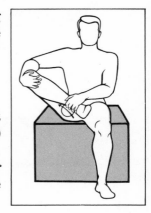

METHOD:

1. Sit down.

2. Grasp the upper side of your right or left ankle (*choose your most painful side*) with your opposite hand in an overhand hold.

3. Place your left or right hand (*your most painful side*) under your knee on the same (*most painful*) side.

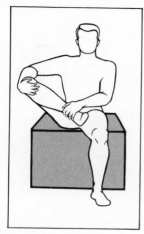

4. Gently press your heel toward your groin and *at the same time* gently pull your knee toward the painful side's shoulder.

5. Hold this position and count from 1001 to 1010. The count may be increased to 1020.

6. Repeat three to five times, once or twice each hour as long as pain relief is being obtained.

Caution: Stop the exercise if pain increases or if numbness or tingling occurs.

MODERATE PAIN, LEVEL 3 CONDITIONING EXERCISES

Continue Exercises #1–#4. Then add the following:

#9 DOUBLE KNEE TO CHEST

This exercise gives a greater *s-t-r-e-t-c-h* to the low back and buttock muscles. It can often be a, very helpful "Feel-Good" Easing Exercise also. If you have knee pain, grasp your hands behind your knees to prevent squeezing them.

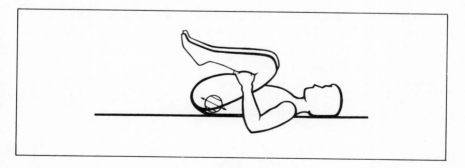

PURPOSE: Generally, to relieve discomfort associated with back pain.

More specifically: to *s-t-r-e-t-c-h* the low back (*lumbosacral*) and buttock (*gluteal*) muscles.

METHOD:

1. Lie on your back on a firm flat surface or on the floor. Bend your knees. Rest your feet *flat* on the "floor." (*A small pillow may be used under your head for comfort.*)

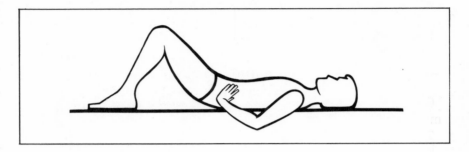

2. Do a mild pelvic tilt.

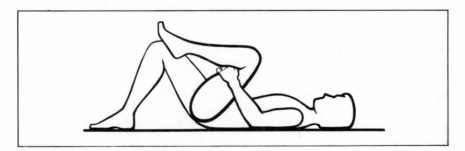

3. Keeping your knee bent, slowly raise the leg that is on your most painful side *first*. Then raise your opposite leg to join it.

4. Release the pelvic tilt.

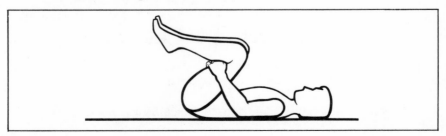

5. Grasp just behind your knees with both hands. Pull your knees gradually toward your chest until you feel a mild *s-t-r-e-t-c-h* in your lower back or at the back of your hip.

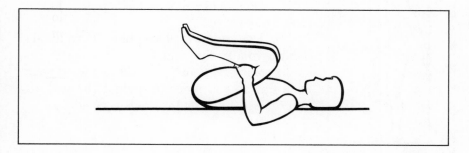

6. Hold and count out loud: 1001, 1002, and 1003. Breathe normally.

7. Relax.

8. Carefully lower your "good" leg first (*remember to keep your knee bent*) to the starting position. Then lower your other leg with your knee bent.

9. Relax.

10. Repeat three to five times, twice daily; once or twice hourly if it helps to relieve your back pain; and once daily on your maintenance program.

#10 WALL SLIDE, 30-DEGREE ANGLE

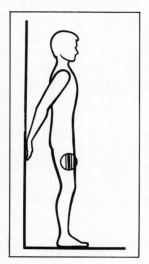

This exercise helps to strengthen the thigh (*quadriceps*) muscles and the buttock (*gluteal*) muscles to permit squatting with ease, or sitting and arising from chairs with good control.

PURPOSE: Generally, to condition the thigh (*quadriceps*) muscles for ease in squatting.

More specifically: to strengthen the quadriceps muscles.

METHOD:

1. Stand with your back a foot away from the wall and your feet about a foot apart.

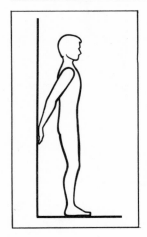

2. Do a mild pelvic tilt. Keep your knees slightly bent.

3. For support, place one or both hands behind you on the wall.

4. Maintain your pelvic tilt and keep your back flat as you place it against the wall (*a helpful position for prolonged standing*).

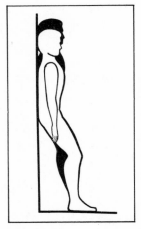

5. By increasing the bend in your knees, slowly slide down the wall until your thighs make a 30-degree angle with the wall.

6. Hold the knee-bent position for 10 counts initially.

7. Slide back up the wall.

8. Repeat, gradually increasing the time of your hold.

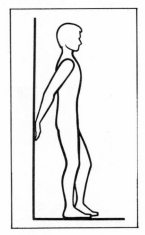

9. Use your hands for support to push, and step away from the wall.

10. Relax.

11. Increase the count gradually to 40 seconds. Gradually increase the angle of your thighs until you can assume a "sitting" position with your back against the wall, without a seat, and hold it for 40 seconds.

12. Do this exercise twice daily.

#11 QUADRICEPS SET (SINGLE STRAIGHT LEG RAISE)

This exercise can be substituted for the Wall Slide 30-Degree Angle to help strengthen the leg muscles when standing is difficult or painful because of foot, ankle, knee, or hip problems.

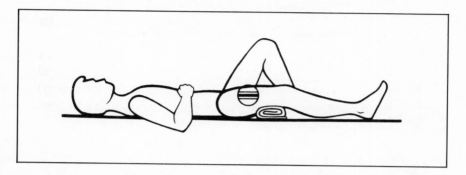

PURPOSE: Generally, to condition the thigh (*quadriceps*) muscles for ease in squatting and arising.

More specifically: to protect the knee while strengthening quadriceps muscles (*isometric*) and building endurance (*isotonic*).

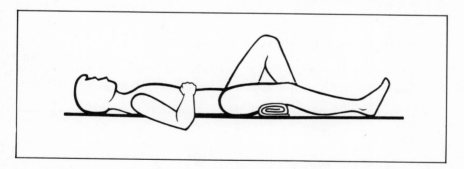

METHOD:

1. Lie on your back with both knees bent and your feet *flat* on a firm flat surface or on the floor.

2. Place a towel-roll or pillow under your right thigh just above the back of your knee. Keep your arms at your sides or on your stomach.

3. Do a mild pelvic tilt.

4. Straighten your right leg. Keep your left leg bent.

5. Press the back of your right thigh down into the towel or pillow as firmly as possible, and pull your right kneecap toward

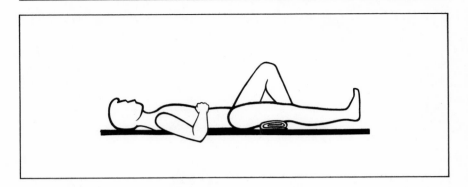

your thigh to tighten your quadriceps muscles. DO NOT ARCH YOUR BACK.

6. Try to increase your effort with each count as you hold and count out loud from 1001 to 1006.

7. Relax, and bend your right leg. Place your foot flat on the floor.

8. Repeat the exercise with a towel or pillow under your left thigh, pressing the left thigh firmly into the towel or pillow.

9. Repeat two times, twice daily until you are on a maintenance program.

#12 SUPINE HAMSTRING *S-T-R-E-T-C-H*

This exercise helps make it easier to bend at the hips and avoid bending at the waist (*the low back is right on your beltline*).

PURPOSE: to relieve strain on the pelvis and the low back caused by tight leg muscles.

More specifically: to *s-t-r-e-t-c-h* or maintain the length of the hamstring muscles.

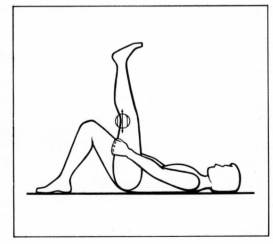

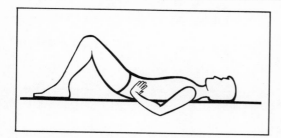

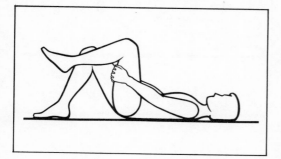

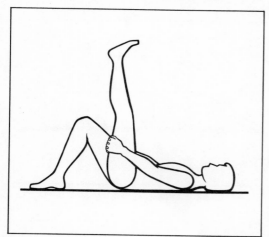

METHOD:

1. Lie down with your knees bent. Do a mild pelvic tilt.

2. Bring your left knee halfway to your chest.

3. Keeping your neck and shoulders relaxed (to avoid neck strain), grasp your left thigh with both hands.

4. Relax the pelvic tilt.

5. Slowly straighten your left knee until you feel a *s-t-r-e-t-c-h* at the back of your knee. Keep your left foot relaxed.

6. Hold and count out loud from 1001 to 1006. DO NOT HOLD YOUR BREATH.

7. Relax.

8. Bend your left knee and return your foot to the starting position.

9. Repeat the exercise by slowly bringing your right knee toward your chest. Grasp your right thigh with both hands and straighten the knee until you feel a *s-t-r-e-t-c-h* at the back of your knee.

10. Repeat three to five times, twice daily until you are on a maintenance program.

#13 BEGINNING PELVIC ROTATION

This exercise can help relieve pain on one side of your lower back or buttocks.

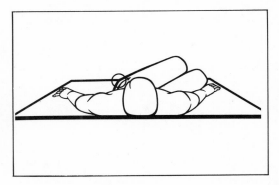

PURPOSE: Generally, to *s-t-r-e-t-c-h* the low back and the hip muscles in a diagonal pattern.

More specifically: to relieve hip and back stiffness and discomfort in order to improve leg and back mobility.

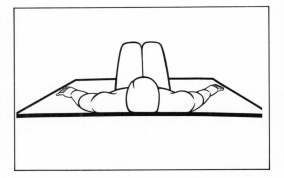

METHOD:

1. Lie on your back on a firm, flat surface or on the floor with both knees bent. Do a mild pelvic tilt.

2. Place both hands at your sides with your palms down and about 18 inches away from your hips.

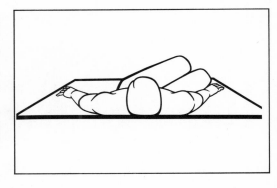

3. Moving both knees together, slowly rotate your hips to your right side as far as you can. You should feel a gentle *s-t-r-e-t-c-h*.

4. Hold and count out loud from 1001 to 1006.

5. Relax.

6. Return to the starting position with both knees bent.

7. Move both legs to the left side as far as you can rotate them. Feel a gentle *s-t-r-e-t-c-h*. Hold, and count from 1001 to 1006.

8. Relax.

9. Return to the starting position with both knees bent.

10. Repeat three to five times, twice daily; or once or twice each hour if it helps relieve your back or buttock pain; and once daily on your maintenance program.

#14 PARTIAL "SIT-UP" (ABDOMINAL ISOMETRIC)

This is a much more strenuous exercise than Exercise #3, Partial "Sit-Up." It gives you the advantage of further strengthening and tightening your abdominal muscles in a sit-up position without straining your back by repeatedly pumping up and down. When you can hold this position for 40 seconds and perform Exercises #1–#4 and #9-#14 with comfort, you are definitely ready for Mild Pain, Level 2 Conditioning Exercises.

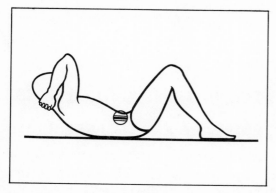

PURPOSE: to strengthen the abdominal muscles in order to help alleviate stress on the back muscles.

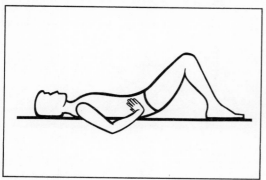

METHOD:

1. Lie on your back on a firm, flat surface or on the floor. Bend your knees. Rest your feet *flat* on the "floor." (*A small pillow may be used under your head for comfort.*)

2. Do a mild pelvic tilt. If possible, hold the tilt throughout the exercise.

3. Grasp your hands at the base of your skull so that your neck is *supported* by your hands. Keep your chin *tucked in* and use your abdominal muscles to slowly raise your head and shoulders until your shoulder blades no longer touch the floor. DO NOT USE YOUR HANDS OR NECK TO LIFT YOUR SHOULDERS.

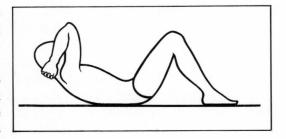

4. Hold and count out loud from 1001 up to 1040 if possible. DO NOT HOLD YOUR BREATH.

5. Return slowly to the starting position.

6. Then relax.

7. Repeat one time, twice daily.

MILD PAIN, LEVEL 2 CONDITIONING EXERCISES

#15 CROSSED HIP ROTATOR *S-T-R-E-T-C-H* (PRETZEL)

This is a good thigh-buttock stretch, but it can cause pain in the thigh, so *only do it if it feels good*. A slight change in the position of the upper leg may help relieve discomfort.

PURPOSE:

1. to *s-t-r-e-t-c-h* the buttock (*gluteal*) and the outer thigh muscles;

2. to help prevent a possible strain when twisting the low back unavoidably.

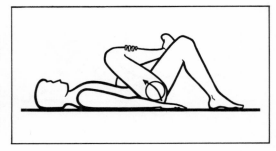

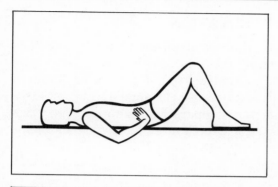

METHOD:

1. Lie on your back on a firm, flat surface or on the floor.

2. Bend both knees and rest your feet *flat* on the "floor."

3. Do a gentle pelvic tilt. Hold the tilt.

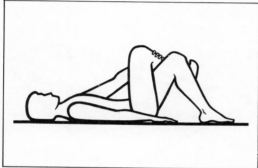

4. Cross your right leg over your left knee.

5. Bring your right knee up toward your chest.

6. Place your left hand around your right knee.

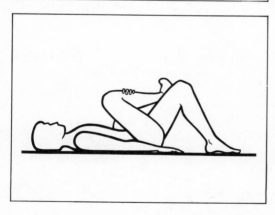

7. Relax your pelvic tilt.

8. Gently pull your right knee toward your left shoulder with your left hand, until you feel a slight *s-t-r-e-t-c-h* in your outer thigh and buttock.

9. Hold this mild *s-t-r-e-t-c-h* and count from 1001 to 1006.

10. Relax. Do a mild pelvic tilt and return to the starting position.

11. Continue the exercise on the opposite side.

12. Repeat three to five times, twice a day, and then once daily on your maintenance program.

Caution: Stop the exercise if pain in the thigh occurs.

#16 ADVANCED PELVIC ROTATION

This exercise stretches the muscles that turn the low back and the hips (*external rotators*). It is also a good pre-athletic warm-up *s-t-r-e-t-c-h*. It is not unusual to get a cracking sound in your back when you do this one because the small facet joints (*see Fig. 9, pg. 14*) can be momentarily separated or gapped. The crack is neither good nor bad, but the stretch often feels good and helps restore mobility to the spine.

PURPOSE: Generally, to increase flexibility in the back and hip muscles and to protect against strain when twisting cannot be avoided.

More specifically:

1. to *s-t-r-e-t-c-h* the hip external rotators and the buttock (*gluteal*) muscles;

2. to *s-t-r-e-t-c-h* the *quadratus lumborum* (the muscles along the back side of your waist) and the *paraspinal* (each side of the spine) muscles.

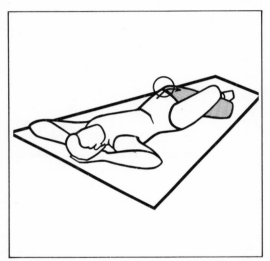

METHOD:

1. Lie flat on your back with your knees bent and your feet resting *flat* on the floor.

2. Clasp your hands behind your head.

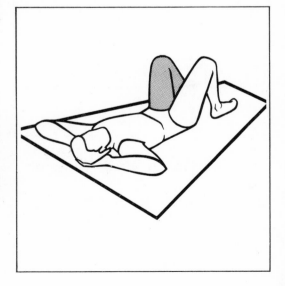

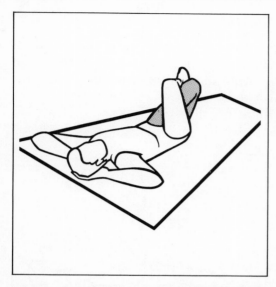

3. Cross your right leg over your left leg; place your right foot on the outside of the left leg *just below* your left knee.

4. Do a gentle pelvic tilt.

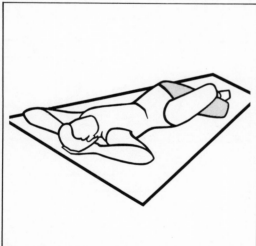

5. Keeping your upper back and shoulders stationary, use your right foot to steadily push your left knee toward the floor on your right side. You should feel a *s-t-r-e-t-c-h* in your left lower back or outer thigh as you try to touch your left knee to the floor.

6. Hold the *s-t-r-e-t-c-h* for a count from 1001 to 1006.

7. Return to the starting position. Relax.

8. Repeat the exercise using your left foot on the outside of your right leg (just below the knee) to push your right knee toward the floor on your left side.

9. Repeat three to five times, twice daily, and once daily on your maintenance program.

#17 SUPINE HAMSTRING *S-T-R-E-T-C-H*
(OPPOSITE LEG STRAIGHT)

This exercise stretches the hamstrings further, and also stretches the muscles in the front of the opposite hip.

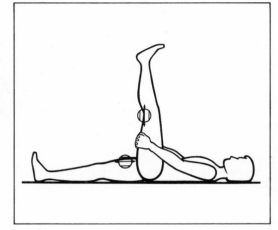

PURPOSE: to *s-t-r-e-t-c-h* the hamstring muscles and thigh flexors on the extended leg and to help maintain hip mobility.

METHOD:

1. Lie down with your knees bent. Do a gentle pelvic tilt. If possible, hold the tilt throughout the exercise.

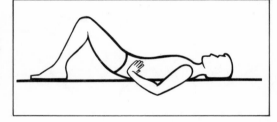

2. Bring your left knee toward your chest and clasp both hands behind your left thigh.

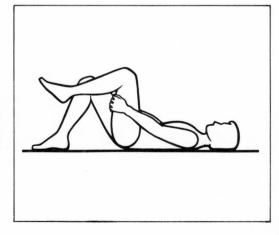

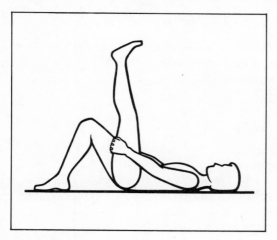

3. Slowly straighten your left knee until you feel a *s-t-r-e-t-c-h* behind the back of your knee. Your foot should be relaxed.

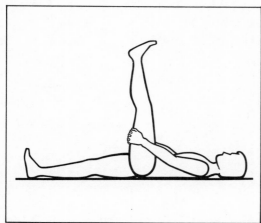

4. Then slide your right (bent) leg until it is straight on the mat. Make an effort to keep your right leg flat and you will feel a *s-t-r-e-t-c-h* on the front of your right leg as well as behind the left knee. Hold and count from 1001 to 1006.

5. Relax. Bend your right knee and then bend your left knee, placing both feet flat on the floor.

6. Repeat the exercise with your *right* knee bent toward your chest and straightening your left leg to the mat.

7. Repeat three to five times, twice daily, until you are on a maintenance program.

#18 CALF *S-T-R-E-T-C-H* (STANDING)

This exercise helps to alleviate tight heel cords (*a common problem in high-heeled shoe wearers*), which pull the knee back, pull on the hamstrings, and strain the back.

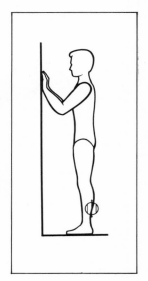

PURPOSE: Generally, to prevent strain while exercising and to relieve cramps in the calves, which may occur at rest or after exercise.

More specifically: to *s-t-r-e-t-c-h* the muscles in the back of the leg (*calf*) so that when walking or squatting the leg and foot work properly.

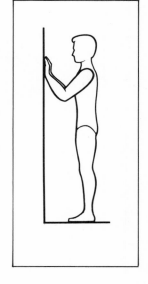

METHOD:

1. Face a wall in your stocking feet with your toes about six inches from the wall.

2. Place the palms of your hands at about shoulder's height on the wall in front of you.

3. Keeping your chin tucked in, do a gentle pelvic tilt.

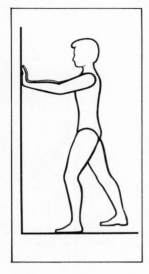

4. Step backward approximately three feet with your right leg.

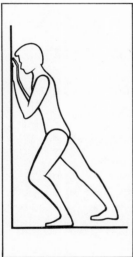

5. Keep your *right heel on the floor* and maintain your pelvic tilt as you bend your arms and *lean* into the wall from your ankle. You should feel a *s-t-r-e-t-c-h* in your lower calf.

6. Count from 1001 to 1006.

7. Return to the starting position.

8. Relax.

9. Repeat the exercise—this time, step back with your left leg.

10. Repeat three to five times, twice daily, and once daily on your maintenance program.

#19 WALL SLIDE REPETITIONS

This exercise is a good way to relieve back strain after prolonged sitting (*as in a movie*) or standing (*waiting to get into the movie*). Doing this repeatedly twenty to forty times is a vigorous aerobic conditioner and an excellent pre-ski workout. BE SURE AND GET YOUR PHYSICIAN'S OKAY BEFORE PERFORMING THIS EXERCISE RAPIDLY AND AEROBICALLY.

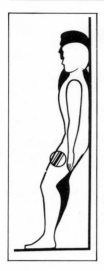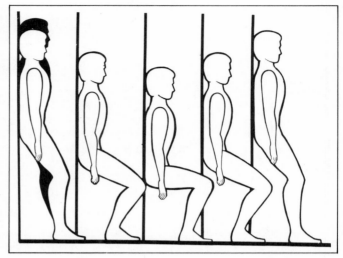

PURPOSE:
1. Generally, to condition the muscles in your legs for ease in squatting and arising;
2. to serve as a back-protected general heart and muscle conditioner (*aerobic exercise*).

More specifically: to strengthen the thigh (*quadriceps*) muscles.

METHOD:
1. Stand with your back a foot away from the wall and your feet about a foot apart.
2. Do a mild pelvic tilt. Keep your knees slightly bent.
3. Place one or both hands behind you on the wall for support.
4. Maintain your tilt and keep your back flat as you place it against the wall (*also a helpful position for any prolonged standing*).
5. By increasing the bend in your knees, slowly *slide* down the wall until your thighs make a 90-degree angle with the wall.
6. Maintain your mild pelvic tilt. Slide back up the wall.
7. Repeat wall slides up and down, as rapidly as possible, three to five times. If needed, place a chair in front of you for balance.
8. As you step away from the wall, maintain your pelvic tilt.
9. Relax.
10. Repeat two times per day for leg conditioning or do twenty to forty repetitions two times a day for aerobic conditioning.

#20 QUADRUPED (CAT BACK)

This exercise helps to limber up the lower back. If you've been very careful to keep your back straight and flat, and are unable to get a good stretch with the Knee to Chest exercise (#2 and #9), the "Cat Back" can help loosen your lower back. BE CAREFUL NOT TO FORCE THE MOTION.

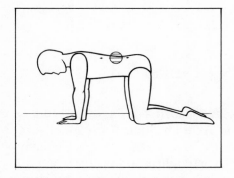

PURPOSE: to s-t-r-e-t-c-h mid- and lower back muscles and to increase back mobility.

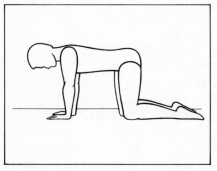

METHOD:

1. Do a mild pelvic tilt. Hold the tilt as you get down on your hands and knees. If necessary, adjust so that your hands are under your shoulders and your knees are under your hip joints.

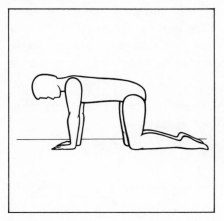

2. Hold your chin in. Look down at the floor. Do a mild pelvic tilt and slowly round your back as high as possible. You should feel a mild s-t-r-e-t-c-h in your mid back.

3. Hold this "cat back" position and count from 1001 to 1006.

4. Relax but DO NOT ALLOW YOUR BACK TO SWAY.

5. Repeat three to five times, two times a day.

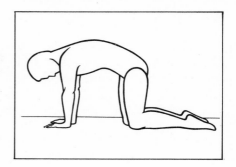

#21 QUADRUPED (HANDS AND KNEES) SINGLE ARM RAISE

This exercise, together with #22 (Quadruped Single Leg Raise) and #23 (Quadruped Contralateral Arm and Leg Raise), helps to condition the muscles of the entire back. This is particularly important in patients susceptible to osteoporosis, because the pull of these muscles on the skeleton helps maintain bone calcium. This exercise looks easy, but it can also easily increase back pain. IT SHOULD NOT BE ATTEMPTED UNTIL BACK PAIN HAS BEEN INFREQUENT AND MINIMAL IN INTENSITY FOR AT LEAST ONE MONTH. A more vigorous variation of this exercise can be done with weights (1 to 5 pounds) on the wrists and ankles, or by lying prone with pillows under the abdomen, but THIS SHOULD ONLY BE ATTEMPTED UNDER THE SUPERVISION OF A PHYSICIAN OR PHYSICAL THERAPIST.

Sequence: Initially, try Exercise #21 holding one time for six counts. If you have done this for two days without any problems, repeat it twice for six counts, and then do it twice daily for a week. After one week, add Exercise #22 and proceed in the same manner. Wait two more weeks before adding Exercise #23, and do so only if all is going well. In Exercise #23, you can gradually increase to twenty counts in each position, repeating them twice and doing the exercise twice daily.

PURPOSE: to strengthen the shoulder blades and the upper back in a back-protected position.

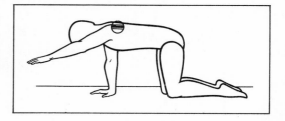

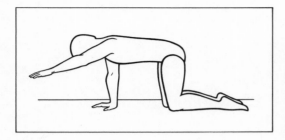

METHOD:

1. Do a mild pelvic tilt. Hold the tilt as you get down on your hands and knees. If necessary, adjust so that your hands are under your shoulders and your knees are under your hip joints.

2. Hold your chin in. Look down at the floor. Do a mild pelvic tilt and raise your left arm approximately 12 inches off the floor. (*Keep the arm below shoulder height.*)

3. Hold and count out loud from 1001 to 1006.

4. Put your arm down.

5. Relax but DO NOT ALLOW YOUR BACK TO SWAY.

6. Repeat this exercise raising your right arm as instructed above.

7. See text above for sequence repetitions.

Caution: Stop the exercise if back or leg pain increases.

#22 QUADRUPED SINGLE LEG RAISE

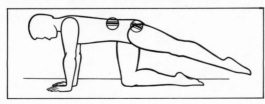

PURPOSE: to strengthen the buttock, posterior thigh, and lower back muscles in a back-protected position.

METHOD:

1. Hold your chin in. Look down at the floor. Do a mild pelvic tilt, and raise your left leg approximately 3 to 4 inches off the floor. Avoid extension of your back.

2. Hold the raised leg and count from 1001 to 1006.

3. Put your leg down.

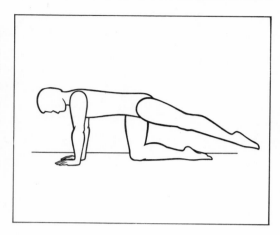

4. Relax. DO NOT ALLOW YOUR BACK TO SWAY.

5. Repeat the exercise, raising your right leg as instructed above.

6. See Exercise #21 for sequence repetitions.

Caution: Stop the exercise if back or leg pain increases.

#23 QUADRUPED CONTRALATERAL ARM AND LEG RAISE

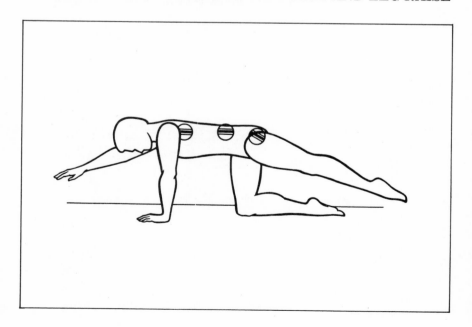

PURPOSE:

1. to simultaneously strengthen the muscles on the opposite sides of the spine;

2. to improve coordination and control for reaching during household and athletic activities.

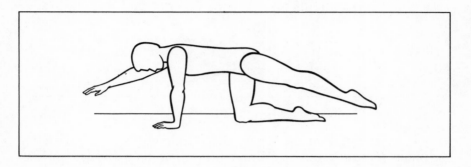

METHOD:

1. Hold your chin in. Look down at the floor. Do a mild pelvic tilt, and raise your left leg approximately 3 to 4 inches off the floor. Raise your right arm 12 inches off the floor.

2. Hold and count out loud from 1001 to 1006.

3. Relax WITHOUT SWAYING YOUR BACK.

4. Repeat the exercise, raising your right leg and your left arm as instructed above.

5. See Exercise #21 for sequence repetitions.

Caution: Stop the exercise if back or leg pain increases.

MINIMAL PAIN, LEVEL 1 CONDITIONING EXERCISES

#24 PUSH-UPS (KNEES BENT)

When your back is strong enough for you to do one push-up without arching your back, you are ready for this exercise. If you have painful arms, shoulders, or knees, back off until they're better. This exercise can be used as an aerobic conditioner, and it strengthens the arms as well as the back. It is easier than the customary push-up with the knees straight (Exercise #25). Many women who cannot do the conventional push-up can perform very well in the Knees Bent version. You should be able to do twenty repetitions of the Knees Bent push-up before trying the Knees Straight version (Exercise #25).

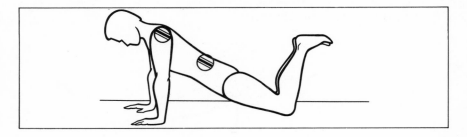

PURPOSE:

1. to strengthen the arms, the shoulders, and the back for optimum strength and coordination in vigorous activities such as lifting, pushing, and pulling;

2. to use as part of an overall aerobic program

3. to maintain proper bone calcium metabolism.

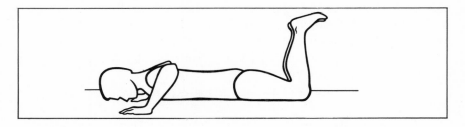

METHOD:

1. Lie flat on your stomach on a mat or a well-padded carpet, with the palms of your hands under your shoulders.

2. Bend your knees.

3. Do a gentle pelvic tilt.

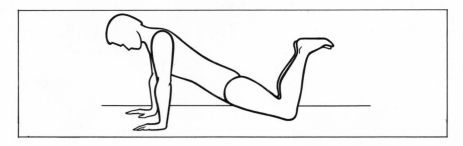

4. Keep your back flat and your chin tucked in as you "push-up" by straightening your arms.

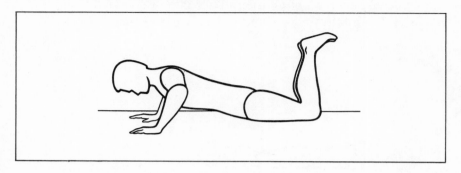

5. Use your arms to slowly lower yourself almost to the floor and, without stopping, repeat the exercise, gradually working your way up to twenty repetitions.

6. After you are able to do the exercise slowly (*this comes with practice*), repeat the push-up (*with your knees bent*) as rapidly as possible—but always remain *in good control*. DO NOT ATTEMPT TO INCREASE THE TEMPO OF THE EXERCISE UNTIL YOU ARE ABLE TO DO IT SLOWLY. BE SURE AND GET YOUR PHYSICIAN'S OKAY BEFORE PERFORMING THE EXERCISE RAPIDLY AND AEROBICALLY.

7. Repeat the exercise twenty times, once per day.

#25 PUSH-UPS (KNEES STRAIGHT)

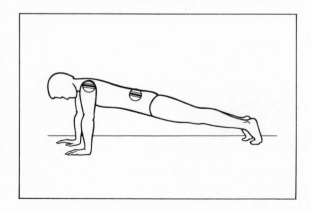

PURPOSE:

1. to use your body weight to strengthen the arms, the

shoulders, and the back for optimum strength and coordination in vigorous activities such as lifting, pushing, and pulling;

2. to use as part of an overall aerobic program;

3. to maintain proper bone calcium metabolism.

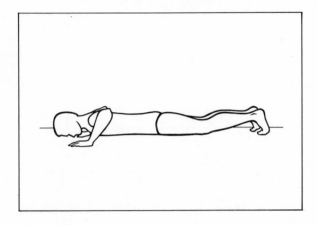

METHOD:

1. Lie flat on your stomach on a mat or a well-padded carpet, with the palms of your hands under your shoulders.

2. Do a gentle pelvic tilt.

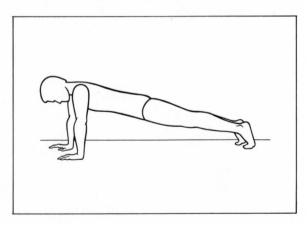

3. Keep your back flat, chin tucked in, and knees straight as you "push-up" by straightening your arms.

4. Use your arms to slowly lower yourself almost to the floor and, without stopping, repeat the exercise, gradually working your way up to twenty repetitions.

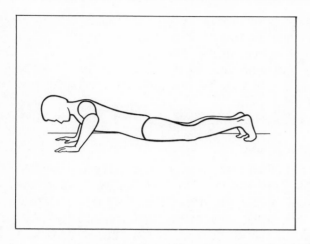

5. After you are able to do the exercise slowly (*this comes with practice*), repeat the push-up as rapidly as possible—but always remain *in good control*. DO NOT ATTEMPT TO INCREASE THE TEMPO OF THE EXERCISE UNTIL YOU ARE ABLE TO DO IT SLOWLY. BE SURE AND GET YOUR PHYSICIAN'S OKAY BEFORE PERFORMING THIS EXERCISE RAPIDLY AND AEROBICALLY.

6. Repeat the exercise twenty times, twice per day.

Caution: Stop the exercise if you begin to feel weak.

This is the last of the series of formal exercises. You are now ready for your "Feel-Good" Easing Exercises, Maintenance Program (*see Chapter 27*), Five-Minute Back Saver (*see Chapter 28*), and Back to Sports (*see Chapter 29*).

THE "FEEL-GOOD" EASING EXERCISES

Nothing succeeds like success itself. If an exercise succeeds in relieving discomfort, it's a sure winner. These "Feel-Good" Easing Exercises often do just that. There's no sure solution or exercise for every problem or back pain, but some or all of these exercises may prove invaluable in easing your pain, lessening the need for pain relieving medications, and helping you keep active and feeling good!

1. When your back feels a little tight, or when there's a slight twinge or catch at times, try:

a. Basic Pelvic Tilt (Exercise #1)

b. Single Knee to Chest (Exercise #2)

c. Double Knee to Chest (Exercise #9)
Some people find just holding in this position for 10 to 20 seconds or holding and gently rocking on their backs can help relieve low back pain.

2. If it's more comfortable leaning back than bending forward, try:

a. Press-Ups (Exercise #5)
If you've done it before and know it helps, try ten repetitions hourly. Do this exercise in bed before arising, or hourly if you are at Severe Pain, Level 4 or Moderate Pain, Level 3, but ONLY IF YOU'VE BEEN EVALUATED AND INSTRUCTED UNDER YOUR DOCTOR'S SUPERVISION. This is a good exercise to do on the floor after your other "Do-Good" Exercises, and it is useful for all pain levels.

b. Back Bends, Standing (Exercise #6)
Do it only if you've done it safely before. This is a good exercise to prevent strain from prolonged sitting, standing, and stooping, and it is useful for Moderate Pain, Level 3 to Minimal Pain, Level 1.

3. If it's sore on one side or in one buttock, try:

a. Knee Back (Lying and Sitting) (Exercises #7 and #8)

b. Beginning Pelvic Rotation (Exercise #13)

c. Crossed Hip Rotator *S-t-r-e-t-c-h* (Pretzel) (Exercise #15)

d. Advanced Pelvic Rotation (Exercise #16)

27.

THE MAINTENANCE

EXERCISE

PROGRAM

When you have reached the level of back conditioning suitable to your customary activities, you have probably completed Moderate Pain, Level 3 conditioning exercises and are performing Mild Pain, Level 2 and Minimal Pain, Level 1 conditioning exercises on a twice daily basis (*see Chapter 26*). If you have been at your highest level of exercise for a month, and if you have only mild or minimal back pain or sciatic pain, you are ready to cut back to a once-a-day exercise program to keep your back in shape. Remember, this is not an athletic training or aerobic conditioning regimen (those are ideally performed on alternate days), so a daily routine is what you need.

This maintenance program may include special emphasis (more repetitions or prolonged holding time) on certain stretching or strengthening exercises in addition to the overall back conditioning exercise program.

The program consists of a sequence of exercises, starting with stretches, primarily done lying down but followed by kneeling and, finally, standing exercises.

The maintenance program should include Exercises #1, #2, #9, and #14 to #20 if they have already been incorporated into your daily exercise regimen. The program should end with five to ten repetitions of Exercise #6 (if back bends have been part of your treatment), so that you can start your day out right.

For a sedentary person at a mild pain level, the following is an example of a typical exercise maintenance program.

SAMPLE PROGRAM—MILD PAIN, LEVEL 1, SEDENTARY		
EXERCISE #	NAME	REPETITIONS/ HOLDS
1	Basic Pelvic Tilt	3
2	Single Knee to Chest	3
3 or 4	Partial "Sit-Up" or Knee Push with Chair	hold up to 40 seconds
9	Double Knee to Chest	3
12	Supine Hamstring *S-t-r-e-t-c-h*	2
13	Beginning Pelvic Rotation	3
10	Wall Slide 30-Degree Angle	hold up to 40 seconds
11	Quadriceps Set	5

If you have mild back pain and are doing almost everything except for heavy work or vigorous athletics, your maintenance program should resemble the following.

SAMPLE PROGRAM—MILD PAIN, LEVEL 1, ACTIVE		
EXERCISE #	NAME	REPETITIONS/ HOLDS
1	Basic Pelvic Tilt	2
9	Double Knee to Chest	3
12	Supine Hamstring *S-t-r-e-t-c-h*	2
14	Partial "Sit-Up"	40-second hold
15	Crossed Hip Rotator *S-t-r-e-t-c-h* (Pretzel)	2
16	Advanced Pelvic Rotation	3
17	Supine Hamstring *S-t-r-e-t-c-h* (Opposite Leg Straight)	2
23	Quadruped Contralateral Arm and Leg Raise	40-second hold
18	Calf *S-t-r-e-t-c-h* (Standing)	1 on each side
19	Wall Slide Repetitions	20
6	Back Bends, Standing	5

If you have minimal back pain and want to further condition your back, you'll add Exercise #25, Push-Ups (Knees Straight) for twenty repetitions before standing up for Exercise #18, and then finish off with Exercise #6. In the event of a relapse while you are on your maintenance program, revert back to a gentle version of the Severe Pain, Level 4 and Moderate Pain, Level 3 exercises (*see Chapter 26*) and any of the exercises that have proven helpful under the "Feel Good" Easing Exercise list (*see pg. 263*). Gradually increase the frequency and vigor of your exercises, progressing through all of your exercises until you can resume a maintenance program.

The whole maintenance exercise program should be completed in less than 10 minutes before you leave the house in the morning. If your alarm didn't go off, you can do it when you get home at night. This small investment of *back* time can pay *back* large dividends and accumulate a treasure of *back* savings.

EXERCISES WHEN SEATED

If you are stuck in a seat for a long trip, or at your desk, or wherever, you may want to do some extra back maintenance exercises to prevent back strain. These exercises, performed every 20 to 30 minutes if possible, can help maintain your back in good shape.

1. Support yourself with your hands on the chair arms. Remain seated and alternately raise and lower each knee five times.

2. Put your hands on your knees and keep your back straight. Using your hands for support, lean forward, stretching, and count to five. Squeeze your buttocks and return to the sitting posture by pushing with your hands and pulling up with your back muscles. Pull from *below upwards*, one vertebra at a time. Repeat this exercise three times.

3. Raise one foot onto the seat of your chair. Grasp the front of the ankle with one hand, cradle the knee with the other hand, and then stretch your knee toward your shoulder for a count of 5 to 10 (*see Exercise #8, pg. 236*).

28.

THE FIVE-MINUTE

BACK SAVER

The Five-Minute Back Saver is an exercise sequence designed to gradually warm your muscles so that they can then be more easily stretched. The Five-Minute Back Saver relieves the night's accumulated muscle and ligament tightness and tension so that your back will move more freely and comfortably and be less susceptible to strain during the day. The Five-Minute Back Saver is performed on a pad or rug on the floor, or on a firm mattress, and before breakfast (or after, if it's a light breakfast). Choose a warm place, or at least one that is not drafty, and wear loose clothing, if needed, to stay warm.

This is an overall stretching-strengthening routine that helps you start out the day with your Back First. The Five-Minute Back Saver is also an excellent warm-up and cool-down for before and after athletics. Be sure that you can perform each of the exercises *comfortably before* you try the whole routine, and eliminate those that cause too much discomfort.

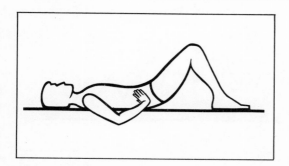

I. Lie down in the Basic Pelvic Tilt (*see Exercise #1, pg. 225*) position. Do an easy one (*just checking*).

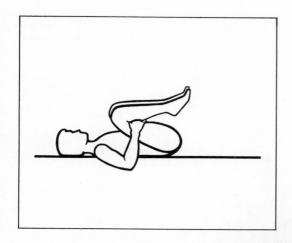

II. Do a Double Knee to Chest slowly (*see Exercise #9, pg. 237*). Hold onto your thighs and kick your feet slightly upward so as to rock on your back for three to five brisk repetitions. Keep your knees bent and return your feet to the floor.

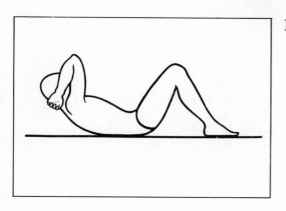

III. Assume the Partial "Sit-Up" posture with your knees bent (*see Exercise #14, pg. 245*). Grasp your hands behind your head or neck and raise your shoulder blades off the floor (*this strengthens the abdominal muscles*).

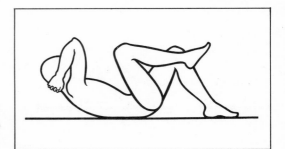

Counts 1 & 2
On the first two counts, bring your right knee to your chest, and then, keeping the right heel just off the floor, straighten the right leg fully so that the leg is just above the floor. This is the *starting* position.

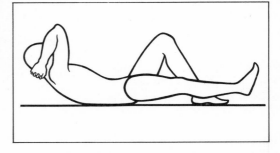

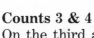

Counts 3 & 4
On the third and fourth counts, keep your right leg straight and raise it vertically overhead, and then lower the leg to return to the starting position (*heel off the floor*). This is called the vertical leg raise.

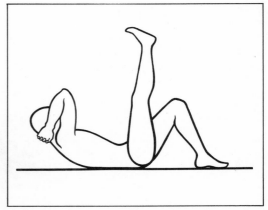

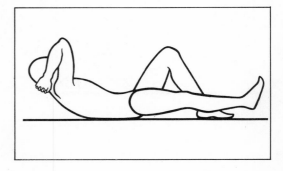

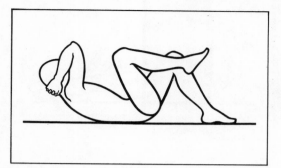

Count 5
Bring your right knee to
your chest and . . .

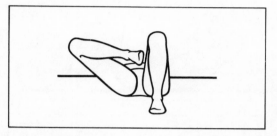

Count 6
Rotate your bent leg out-
ward into a frog-leg po-
sition. Keep the knee
and leg as horizontal as
possible while straight-
ening the leg. Turn the
foot up (*vertically*) when
you are again at the starting position.

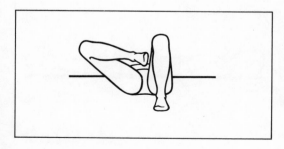

Count 7
Return the knee to the
chest, keeping the knee
and the leg in the frog-
leg position and in the
horizontal plane and . . .

Count 8
Straighten the leg, keep-
ing it just off the floor,
and return it to the starting position.

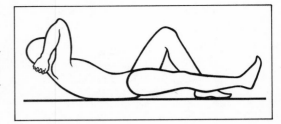

Count 9
Repeat the vertical leg
raise with the knee
straight and . . .

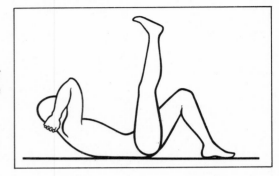

Count 10
Bend the knee and place
the foot back on the floor
(*as in Exercise #14, pg.
245*).

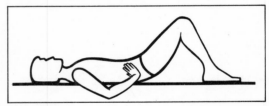

    Repeat the entire series with the opposite leg, and then
repeat the sets (*a set is one time with your left leg and one time
with your right leg*) at an increasingly more rapid tempo until ten
full sets are completed. (*Now you are getting warm.*)

IV. Lower your head
and shoulders to the
floor. Hold a 6-
second Quadriceps
Set (*see Exercise
#11, pg. 241*) on each
side, with as much
effort as you can
possibly make. (*This
strengthens the legs
for squatting.*)

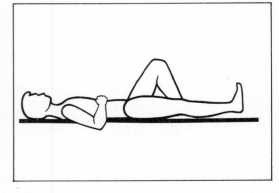

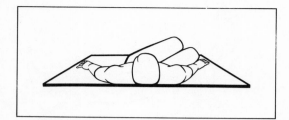

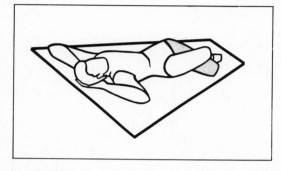

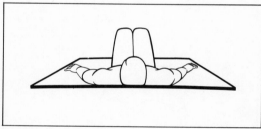

V. Place your legs in the Partial "Sit-Up" position while keeping your head and shoulders on the floor. Do a Beginning Pelvic Rotation (*see Exercise #13, pg. 244*) slowly to each side. (*You're just checking.*)

VI. Do an Advanced Pelvic Rotation (*see Exercise #16, pg. 248*) slowly to each side (*a little more checking*).

VII. Do another Advanced Pelvic Rotation to the right. Hold for a count of 1 and 2.

VIII. Return to the Partial "Sit-Up" position (*head and shoulders on floor*).

IX. Cross your legs on the opposite side, do a Basic Pelvic Tilt, and repeat the Advanced Pelvic Rotation on the left side (*you're getting the kinks out*).

X. Do five full sets to each side.

XI. Roll over onto your abdomen and do five Press-Ups (*see Exercise #5, pg. 232*), keeping your pelvis on the floor. (*This can keep the disks from bulging back.*)

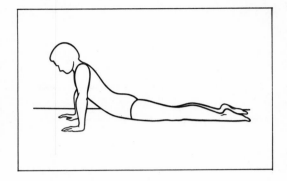

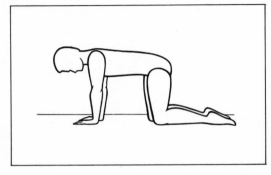

XII. Assume the Quadruped (*hands and knees*) position.

XIII. Arch your back and hold a "Cat Back" posture (*see Exercise #20, pg. 255*). Keeping your hands in place, sit back onto your heels. (This will s-t-r-e-t-c-h the lower spine.)

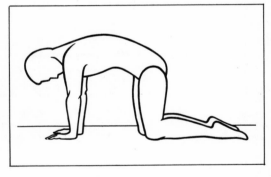

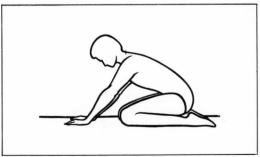

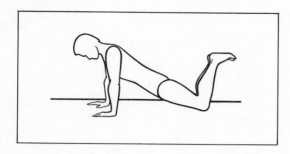

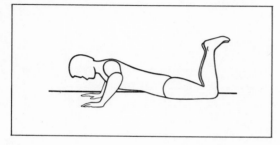

XIV. Do a Push-Up (Knees Bent) (*see Exercise #24, pg. 259*), or if you can without arching your back, do a full Push-Up (Knees Straight) (*see Exercise #25, pg. 261*), and hold with your elbows bent for a count of 20 to 25. Alternatively, do five to ten slow Push-Ups (Knees Bent or Knees Straight) under full control. (*This strengthens the arms and shoulders.*)

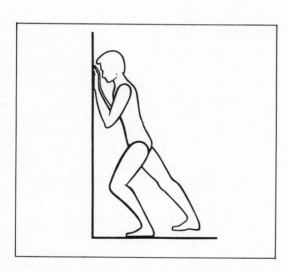

XV. Stand up with your feet at shoulder width, toes pointed slightly in, and *s-t-r-e-t-c-h* each heel cord (*see Exercise #18, pg. 252*).

You've done your exercises. Good! Take a moment to reflect on the Four Back Words: BACK FIRST, BACK FLAT, BACK STRAIGHT, and BACK LAST. Remember, *Feet First and Face It!* Now you're ready to start the day.

29.

BACK

TO SPORTS

PLAY BACK

There are many reasons to exercise, and most of us participate in recreational sports because we enjoy them, but if you have a back problem, your first exercise need is for therapeutic exercise. These exercises are designed to relieve muscle spasm and pain, and also to stretch muscles and ligaments that have become tight from lack of use or from improper use. Strengthening is needed to allow adequate strength for posture and for performance of daily activities without causing strain. Finally, warm-up and cooldown prophylactic therapeutic exercises are prescribed to prepare the body for more vigorous activities and to relieve tensions in muscles after strenuous exertion. Some of these exercises, once structured into a habitual routine, can be a source of comfort. Most former patients look forward to them with pleasure and the knowledge that they will feel better when they are stretched out and limbered up. Some get a meditationlike benefit from the exercise ritual in much the way that yoga or Tai Chi seems to work. In fact, there are close parallels in the Iyengar school of Hatha yoga to many of the back exercises. For many of those patients who enjoy yoga, the appropriate yoga exercise can be substituted in their maintenance routine.

One of the most popular forms of exercise today cannot be strictly construed as recreational. This is aerobic exercise or exercises that use a great deal of energy and are designed to achieve endurance fitness. The hope that heart attacks and strokes will be prevented and a long and healthy life assured lies very close to the surface for many committed aerobic exercisers. There is also some evidence that sustained grueling physical activity has a numbing effect on nervous tension. Possibly this sensation comes about by the release of the body's own morphinelike endorphins. For some, the relentless pursuit of the ultimate physical stress, even to the point of pain, becomes the goal of exercise, with a sense of elation, at a point near exhaustion (the runner's "high"), as the desired reward.

There is, in fact, no indisputable scientific evidence that aerobic exercise in any form prevents heart attacks or strokes. There is good evidence that excessive physical stress, even in well conditioned athletes, often leads to musculoskeletal strain, and in this regard the back is very vulnerable. So why exercise? Because it is fun and it makes us feel good! Yes, the criteria for Back to Sports should be enjoyable exercise that we can do in a manner that entails minimum risk for our backs.

THE WARM-UP AND COOL-DOWN

They walk horses, don't they? Yes, and they shoot them, too, but it's clearly better to walk on and off of your favorite sport activity than to stiffen up and get a "shot" in the back. The principle of warm-up exercises is that exercises increase local muscle metabolism and heat. Warm muscles stretch more easily and are protected against strain. Professional pitchers always keep their pitching arms protected and warm, and you should be sure that your muscles are warm and stretched before engaging in any sport. A good pre-athletic injury-prevention program consists of walking and walk-jogging for three to five minutes; then stretch by going through your maintenance exercises (*see Chapter 27*) and any additional stretches required by your sport. If you're a swimmer, a few minutes of walking or treading in deep water (if it's warm enough) before you swim, combined with stretching in the water, is also a good precautionary warm-up.

The cool-down lets the circulation gently clear out irritating by-products of exercise metabolism. This helps avoid muscle spasm and cramps. The three to five minute walk-off followed by your maintenance stretching should do the job—unless you've played too hard and strained your back.

WALK BACK

Walking is a universal source of pleasure. One has to wonder why we search so diligently for the parking space closest to wherever we have to go when a short walk would be a pleasant alternative in the offing. For back pain patients, walking can be an excellent activity for mild physical conditioning and for recreation.

STROLL BACK—MODERATE PAIN, LEVEL 3 WALKING

Good walking shoes are essential. Begin walking short distances and avoid steps. A rule of thumb for a safe initial walk is to select a distance that is roughly one half of what you are *sure* you can do. Listen to your body and make sure you're not getting any *back* talk. Try that short walk, and if that works then go 75% of the distance the next day. If in doubt, stay at the same distance but walk two to three times each day. Then walk the "full" distance. If that is well tolerated, walk a little more briskly the next time. Always rest en route if you feel the need. Remember that a sore foot, ankle, knee, or hip, or a heavy purse, can change your stride and strain your back. So don't neglect any of these problems, and be sure that your shoes give the best support possible for your feet and legs. A power-driven treadmill is an excellent device on which to begin a walking program or to continue one if it is inconvenient to walk outdoors. The power-driven treadmill reduces friction and the jarring that occurs with each step, but it still provides an excellent walking exercise conditioner.

HIKE BACK—MILD PAIN, LEVEL 2 WALKING

Gradually increase the walking distance and tempo. If you're expanding your horizons in walking up and down hills, remember that walking up a slight incline is usually easier on your back than walking downhill because it keeps your back in a slight pelvic tilt position (*see Exercise #1 pg. 225*).

BACK PACKING—MINIMAL PAIN, LEVEL 1 WALKING

Travel light, use a walking stick if hiking over rough terrain, and carry as much around your waist and as little on your back as possible. Don't get over tired! Ask for help in getting your pack on and off—there is no sense ruining an outing at either end by wrestling with your pack. Do not race walk. The hip twisting will get you in the back.

RUN BACK

The committed runner will settle for nothing less than getting *Back into Stride*. Unfortunately, this is not always possible, but since it often is, it's worth a try—go back to running slowly and carefully.

■ *Back First*. Don't return to running until your back has healed or at least your symptoms are minimal, stable, and not aggravated by brisk walking. Warm up before and cool down after every run. Run on a level, firm (but not cement), hard surface, and use well fitted socks and well cushioned running shoes. If your only terrain is up and down hills, run up and then walk briskly down.

■ *Back Flat*. Concentrate on keeping your abdomen tight and with a slight pelvic tilt—this will feel strange, but eventually it comes naturally.

■ *Back Straight*. Lean from the hips and not from the waist, and avoid running downhill because it can cause excessive arch in your back.

■ *Back Last.* Use a *short*, relatively high-stepping stride to take the shock in your feet and legs and away from your back. Bouncing or jumping, particularly stiff-legged, will jar your back. If your shoes begin to scuff at each stride during your run, you are getting tired. Your back will soon be dragging and it may be time to *walk back.* Some runners find that they can get a good workout on a trampoline, but there is a real danger of being thrown off balance and twisting your back with these devices—so be careful, and hold onto a handrail if you decide to try one.

STROKE BACK

Handball, squash, racketball, table tennis, and badminton (if you're serious about it) are best as spectator sports for most back pain patients. If you are going to try a racket sport, follow the precautions for tennis.

TENNIS—THE BACK HAND IS EVERYTHING

■ *Back First.* Back pain should be gone, or minimal and stable, and not aggravated by your exercises, or by vigorous walking. Your maintenance program should have been performed regularly for a month, and your warm-up and cool-down exercises should be part of your regular routine and used faithfully, before and after any sport activity. Any neck, shoulder, arm, hand, hip, knee, ankle, or foot problems should have been cared for, because in compensating for these problems you may have to take more strain in your back. The racket handle should be well fitted and the racket and strings in good shape and not too taut. Tennis shoes should have full tread on their soles. The court should be level, dry, clean, and if possible made of clay. Be fussy—the back you save may be your own. When first resuming tennis, take lessons, practice ground strokes with a steady partner, or use a backboard. Try easy opponents, and start playing doubles before getting into serious singles competition.

■ *Back Flat.* Use a mild pelvic tilt. Keep your knees bent.

■ *Back Straight.* Don't take a shot unless your whole body is in position. Pivot with your feet. Try to return a shot with your racket at shoulder height. Squat for low shots, bending your knees and hips but keeping your back straight. Overhead shots and service should be performed with the ball well in front of you. Wait for the ball to drop and don't arch your back. For a service return, use a semi-squatting stance with your knees and hips well flexed and your back *straight*.

■ *Back Last*. Get in position for each shot—bend your knees and hips and concede the shots you are not ready for—so you can *come back* and win the next point, game, set, match!

GOLF—SWING (FORE!) BACK

Golf is okay as long as you just putt around—and even that can be dangerous if you stay bent over lining up the putt, or if you forget to squat or kneel to place or retrieve the ball.

■ *Back First*. As always.

■ *Back Flat*. A pelvic tilt for putting is essential.

■ *Back Straight*. Bend from your hips and knees—never from your back when setting your tee or lining up your putt.

■ *Back Last*. Not too difficult when putting, but not everyone is content to stay on the putting green or to play miniature golf.

So let's get serious, it's the Back Swing and follow-through that can keep your back in the rough. There is no safe and sure golf swing, but if you are going to get Back in the Swing, here are some Swing-Back tips.

SWING BACK

■ *Back First*. Don't start golfing until you're pain-free or having minimal, stable, or residual discomfort that is not worsened by general exercise or by specific pelvic rotations or other therapeutic exercises. You should have been on your maintenance program for at least a month before beginning golf. Always do your warm-up before and cool-down after each outing on the driving range or fairway.

Use a tee and your short irons at the beginning, and try hitting a small bucket of balls on the driving range the first time around. Take plenty of time between shots and do a few back bends before and after each shot. If all is okay, use your mid-irons next, your long irons, and finally your woods on subsequent trials. Wear your corset the first few times out—just to remind you to use good body mechanics.

■ *Back Flat.* The mild pelvic tilt and tight stomach muscles are essential throughout the swing.

■ *Back Straight.* Kneel or squat to tee up. Use your club for support. Your back swing and follow-through should both be shortened to avoid or at least minimize twisting motion.

■ *Back Last.* Keep your trunk square, using your arms, hips, and legs for rotation. A clean crisp shot is not much of a worry, but a jarring heavy divot can "do it"—so keep your head down and your eye on the ball!

SPORTS TO STAY AWAY FROM

Unless you are a pro, contact sports (football, basketball, soccer) are best avoided. Bowling and baseball are "twisty" and risky out-of-control sports and are best left alone.

SPORTS TO BACK OFF OF

Aerobic dancing typically has many uncontrolled and jerky movements, and it is worse for your back than horseback riding; which is worse than weight lifting (which can be done with proper precautions—*see "Weights and Backs," below*); which is worse than sailing (a taut ship demands a taut back); which is worse than rowing. Needless to say, all of these sports can be tried and will be by some back pain sufferers—but none should be attempted until your back symptoms have abated or stabilized and you have progressed to a Mild Pain, Level 1 maintenance program (*see pg. 266*) for at least a month. Then—start with caution.

It is a good idea to wear your corset at first (if you have one) just to keep you honest and hopefully out of trouble.

SPORTS TO GO BACK TO

If you are in good condition, start back slowly.

Ice skating, if you are in good condition and good at it, is well tolerated, provided you can skate without arching your back. Surprisingly, so is skiing. Stay off of rope tows, and ski only on good snow, under good control, with good safety equipment. Don't ski when tired. A little early apres-ski is better than a late ride back in the Ski Patrol's toboggan. Your safest and best ski back is cross-country skiing.

FISHING

Fishing is not much exercise, but it's a good source of plea-sure. With good body mechanics, it is reasonably safe, unless you're lucky and hook a big one. In fact, fishing is so sedentary that between bites you have to remember to move and to change positions in order to minimize static strains on your back.

■ *Back First.* Remember to watch how you lift the oars or heavy tackle boxes and outboard motors.

■ *Back Straight.* Cast using your arms and legs and hold that pelvic tilt.

■ *Back Straight.* Remember, you are not in trouble fishing unless you catch a fish: Then it is really time for Back Flat, Back Straight, and Back Last. Better take back a fish story than a *back* sorry.

BIKE BACK

Bicycling, like walking and swimming, is one of the best tolerated exercise activities for people with a low back pain background, but it's got to be done right. Doing it right means not overdoing it.

■ *Back First.* Try a stationary bicycle with proper seat and handlebar adjustments. Be sure that the frame is short enough to permit sitting in an upright posture.

■ *Back Flat.* Sit straight—Bike Back Straight—don't bend over to reach the handlebars. Keep the seat low enough so that your knees are slightly bent when the pedal is down and your hips remain level while you are pedaling.

■ *Back Last.* Partially support your body on your arms, and pump with your legs without moving your back. Optimum pedaling is at 60 to 90 RPM (1 RPM equals one full up-down-up stroke on the pedal per minute), so use gears to maintain a steady pedal stroke. Stretch your legs before mounting, and then pedal at 30 to 45 RPM for the first few minutes to warm up. To cool down, reverse the process and do all of the stretches in your maintenance exercise program.

WEIGHTS AND BACKS

Once a low back pain problem has been resolved or stabilized with minimal residual discomfort and a full Minimal Pain, Level 1 exercise regimen has been accomplished (*see pg. 259*), weight work can be resumed *with caution*, always preceded by a standard warm-up and followed by a cool-down (*see pg. 277*). If you think about it, proper weight-lifting techniques are back protective, and the same principles apply to barbells as to cement bags or shopping bags.

■ *Back First.* Avoid exercises that put weights behind your head or cause excessive stretching of your back. Lie on a bench with your hips and knees flexed for bench presses, or stand with your back leaning against the wall (*see Wall Slide Exercises #10 and #19, pp. 239, 253*). Start with low weight loads and few repetitions. Use a corset or "weight lifter's belt" for lumbar support and abdominal compression. Start light, using less than 50 pounds for males and 25 pounds, including barbells and bar, for females. Do no more than eight repetitions of each exercise per day. Work out on alternate days, giving your body a day of rest to recuperate from the strain. Never hold your breath when lifting. Catch your breath between weight-lifting exercises.

■ *Back Flat.* Tightened buttocks and tightened abdominal muscles are essential in all weight lifting.

■ *Back Straight.* Stand close to the bar with your toes beneath it. Squat with your feet flat and your back straight. Lift only to shoulder-level height.

■ *Back Last.* Let your arms and legs do the work. Be in control at all times. The bent knee dead lift is dangerous unless it is done with light weights (where it will serve as a good model for all situations where lifting of heavy objects is unavoidable). If you want to progress to greater loads, go for more repetitions at the current level before proceeding to the next. For Nautilus, all of the above apply. The safest Nautilus machines are the Double Chest Machine Decline Press and the Biceps Machine.

BACK IN THE SWIM

By and large, swimming is the best all-around recreational sport for people with current or past back problems, or with almost any other joint disorder for that matter. Not only is a pool a good place for a pleasant dip on a hot day, or a great place for vigorous safe exercise, but it can also be used as an ideal area for therapeutic exercise. The buoyancy of the water can be supportive, allowing for ease in stretching; or the resistance of the water can be used to work against during strengthening exercises.

A long shallow pool (25 meters is ideal) roughly 3 to 4 feet in depth with a non-slip floor is the perfect environment. Since diving is out, it should have an easy access ladder and/or steps with rails for safe entry and exit.

SWIM BACK—MODERATE PAIN LEVEL 3

At this stage you are probably looking for a hot tub or a warm pool. If you have one at home, be sure that you know how to get in and out safely (*Back First*). You may need to install bars or tub rails so you can support yourself. Getting up from the tub is the trickiest part of this procedure. *Don't slip* (non-skid matting or tiles are essential). If you have no handrails, turn onto your hands and knees and then get up. It may be best to first empty the tub. If you are using a public hot tub, all of the above apply, and it is also a good idea to find out how they sterilize the tub. Check with your local health department on this one.

Water temperature for tub-soaking is best at 98 to 102°F. For general exercises in water, 90 to 95°F is about right. For comfortable swimming, 82°F is about the right temperature.

About 5 to 10 minutes in the water is long enough for a hot soak or an initial swim. Swimming for 30 to 45 minutes makes a good workout.

If you are going to swim, avoid crowded pools; don't run on slippery surfaces to the shower; be sure your locker is placed at a height that is easily accessible; and protect yourself with a robe if necessary to prevent chilling. Always do your dry-land stretches (maintenance exercises) before entering the water (*see Chapter 27*).

■ *Back Flat*. If you are not a strong swimmer, first try walking in waist-deep water, and be sure to hold your pelvic tilt. Thrashing in the water is best saved until you're all well, and then take lessons if you plan to do swimming as your sport. If you can handle walking in the water—add simulated crawl strokes while walking in water of shoulder level. A 3-minute walk with an arm "crawl" motion, or 1 to 2 minutes of treading, makes a good pre-swimming warm-up. Side stroking or floating on your back while sculling with a gentle pelvic tilt are good initial strokes.

■ *Back Straight*. If you can use a snorkel, this will help keep your face down and minimize the tendency for your back to arch. You can use a kick board or flotation vest to position your chest so that you can keep your back flat with a good pelvic tilt. As you get back into swimming, a good crawl stroke is usually well tolerated. Depending on the action of the scissor kick on your back, the side stroke can be even better, especially if you are not a strong swimmer. The next best stroke (if the pool is uncrowded) is the lazy back stroke.

■ *Back Last.* Warm up arms and legs, and cool down while walking or treading in the water for 1 to 2 minutes. Repeat stretches on dry land.

BACK IN THE SWIM—MILD PAIN, LEVEL 2 TO MINIMAL PAIN, LEVEL 1

■ *Back First.* The same precautions still apply. First go through your maintenance stretches and then warm up for 3 to 5 minutes with slow, easy strokes.

■ *Back Flat.* If you are starting your Swim Back Program at this phase, concentrate on your pelvic tilt. As your back becomes stronger and better conditioned, the pelvic tilt will take care of itself.

■ *Back Straight.* The back stroke can be added, and you might be able to ease into the breast stroke, but only when the other strokes are comfortably performed. Snorkeling is fine. Skin diving, which requires hyperflexion of your spine as you go into the dive, requires some caution. Don't rush back to racing turns. The butterfly and diving are out.

■ *Back Last.* Let's face it—your back is just a connector for your arms and legs to propel in the water when you are swimming, so save your back by doing a cool-down of 1 to 2 minutes of easy treading-water or sculling, and then repeat your dry-land stretches, when you are back out of the water.

DANCE BACK

Dancing *under control* can be a most enjoyable recreation, but be sensible! The *twist* is just what it says it is, and jumping, arching movements; jerky movements; and duck walks or splits are out. There's a lot left. So start with a slow beat and a sensible partner on an uncrowded dance floor or in a studio. Don't start until: (1) you are able to do your Mild Pain, Level 2 and half of Minimal Pain, Level 1 conditioning exercises comfortably, (2) you have been on the maintenance program for a month, and (3) the pain is either entirely gone or minimal and stable. You must do your warm-up before and cool-down after each dance session if you want to Dance Back again.

CONCLUSION

Only two things are certain in life: death and taxes. Almost as inevitable is low back pain. Fortunately, most patients with low back pain recover within a few weeks, with or without any treatment. Unfortunately, many of those who suffer these disabling episodes, no matter how short-lived the episode, have not had the opportunity to learn how to deal with them and, more importantly, how to avoid them.

The *good news* is that most back pain is preventable. The *good news* is that recovery from most low back pain can be expedited by learning and employing the strategies in this book that help relieve pain, restore function, and protect against recurrences of low back pain. *Good News for Bad Backs* is a valuable guidebook for you now if you are suffering from back pain, and it will be a ready resource for you to use if a need should arise at a future time.

It has been said that ignorance is no excuse under the law. It is certainly true that ignorance of back protection, and the assaults that we make on our backs will not be forgiven for long by our backs. We can excuse our ignorance if there is no opportunity to learn. *Good News for Bad Backs* was written so you could have the opportunity to learn how your back works and how you can work to keep the superbly engineered machinery of your back working tirelessly and painlessly on your behalf.

INDEX

*(Page numbers in **boldface** refer to illustrations)*